The Feel Good Handbook

Annie Costa

A survival guide for anyone who suffers from: asthma, migraine headaches, chronic fatigue syndrome, stomach, digestive or intestinal distress, heart, lung, skin or prostrate conditions.

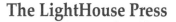

The LightHouse Press

The Feel Good Handbook

Printed in the United States of America.
First printing; January 1998.

ISBN number: 0-9662169-9-7

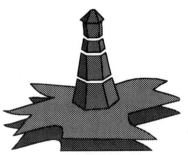

To Order More Copies
of This Book: Call toll-free
888-298-5100.

Or write to:
The LightHouse Press
3555 South El Camino Real, #301
San Mateo, CA 94403

Visit us on the WEB!
www.thelighthousepress.com
www.msgfree.com

ACKNOWLEDGEMENTS

My first exposure to the sources of MSG came from NO MSG, the *National Organization Mobilized to Stop Glutamates*. They in turn introduced me to the Truth in Labeling Campaign (TLC), who in turn introduced me to the work of Russell L. Blaylock, M.D., Jack and Adrienne Samuels, PhD., Dr. John W. Olney, George R. Schwartz, M.D., and others mentioned throughout this book. All, in some part, played a role in my survival and subsequent renewal through the ordeal of eliminating MSG from my life.

I would encourage you to take a voyage of your own through the materials they bring to the public and contact both TLC and NO MSG and draw your own conclusions. Their work and information has made a dramatic impact on me and my family's well being. We owe our health and happiness to them all.

My sincere appreciation goes out to everyone who is working to understand the impact of excitotoxins and I would ask you personally to support them by joining them in their efforts to educate and support us, especially in the regulation and use of excitotoxins in our food supplies and other consumer products. Contact information is located in the Appendices under Organizations & Support Groups.

I would also like to thank my husband Paul and son Alan for their love, patience and support in the authoring of this book. For trying out recipes and meal plans and working as a family to change our lives for the better.

A special thank you goes out to my dear friends and the professionals that helped with information, recipes, editing and proofing this book; ensuring that the content was presented with the utmost integrity and correctness when printed.

Table of Contents

Appendices

This book is dedicated to
J & A
with many thanks
for their support and friendship

"Doc, it always happens when I ..."

One day, for whatever reason, you begin to notice that you get headaches after eating Chinese food. You find your mouth dry; sinuses tight; maybe a prickly sensation in your skin; your gut might be gassy and cramping. This could be anywhere from a mild inconvenience to some extremely uncomfortable symptoms. One thing you know for sure, it happens right after you eat "Chinese".

Concerned, you go to the doctor and he suggests you might have "Chinese Restaurant Syndrome" or CRS; you might be "sensitive" to monosodium glutamate, commonly referred to by consumers as MSG.

"You should avoid eating 'Chinese food' and monosodium glutamate", he states definitively, assuring you that quite a few people are in the same boat as you are. "Nothing to concern yourself over, just watch what you eat!" You pay your bill and go out vowing never to set foot into a "Chinese restaurant" again in your life. You're cured.

Next day, successfully avoiding "Chinese food" for breakfast, you run down to your local sandwich cafe or pop open the refrigerator. You grab a low fat white meat sandwich; slab of tomato and lettuce; low fat mayo and a hearty enriched whole-wheat bun or a great big colorful salad with bottled low-fat buttermilk dressing.

NOTE: *Although most physician's continue to use the term "Chinese Restaurant Syndrome", in July 1995, the Federation of American Societies for Experimental Biology (FASEB), in a study financed by the Federal Drug Administration (FDA), renamed "Chinese Restaurant Syndrome" to "MSG Symptom Complex".*

You look at the labels on the packaged products; no monosodium glutamate here! Must be okay to eat.

Within an hour or so of finishing your meal; poised over the proposal you need to finish or the chores you need to complete; you can't focus on what you are doing. You find yourself "hazy" as if a cold or flu is settling in; and there's that darn headache, dry mouth and throat again. You gulp down a glass of water, force yourself through the project and the symptoms begin to pass . . . whew! Maybe you just "willed" that cold or flu away; must be that positive attitude you try to maintain.

What just happened, really? Chances are you just consumed some form of MSG and had a "sensitivity reaction" to its ingestion.

"I didn't eat 'Chinese food' or monosodium glutamate!" you exclaim. "I read the labels, there wasn't any monosodium glutamate in anything I used! My doctor said to avoid it and I did!"

Well, yes and no. What your doctor said was that you may be suffering from a sensitivity to monosodium glutamate. What he didn't tell you, because he may not have known himself, is that the main ingredient in monosodium glutamate is what is really bothering you. This ingredient is called something entirely different and may not even be clearly mentioned on the labels of the products you used.

What is really bothering you is an amino acid "freed" from protein as a consequence of manufacture. Only products that contain 78% or more of this "freed amino acid", combined with salt, can be called monosodium glutamate. If the product contains less than 78%, it could be labeled using one of more than 30 different names. Most of us consumer-types call it all "MSG". Unfortunately, as consumers, you and I mistakenly may think that only the ingredient monosodium glutamate can cause us adverse reactions, when in reality it is one of its main components, free glutamic acid as a result of manufacture.

Go back and read the label of the luncheon meat, the mayonnaise, the bread, and the buttermilk dressing. Items commonly used in preparing each of these packaged products may be common sources of MSG. People who react to MSG will react to it regardless of the name of the MSG containing ingredient ingested. Here's where the fun begins.

Ever played hide and seek? The rules are pretty simple. Someone hides and someone seeks and you pretty much know that there is one seeker and a specific number of hiders to find. The seeker must close his eyes and count for awhile, allowing the hiders ample time to disappear. Now, in the game I played as a child, we got to open our eyes and look for known targets before they found home base or us. In the game of hide and seek we play with MSG, that's not the case ...

You will need to check your label not only for the ingredient monosodium glutamate, but also other common ingredients that contain MSG that we will call " hidden". We call these "hidden" sources of MSG because the ingredients listed may contain manufactured free glutamic acid, which is never mentioned on the label. The only product on the market that does give us a hint of this is monosodium glutamate.

Some of the hidden MSG will be found in food starch; maltodextrin; hydrolyzed protein, calcium or sodium caseinate; gelatin; soy isolate or soy concentrate; enriched flour; malted barley; yeast; nutritional yeast; autolyzed yeast; and "natural flavors". These additives contain free glutamic acid (MSG).

The three letters M.S.G., together, have become much more than an "acronym" for the ingredient monosodium glutamate. Those three letters, in the lives of consumers, commonly represent ALL free glutamic acid found in products today. If you experience adverse reactions from ingestion of the ingredient monosodium glutamate, it is a good bet that you will also react to any other form of free glutamic acid, if you eat enough of it.

To help those of us who have been told that we are sensitive to monosodium glutamate or MSG, those three letters should be used to represent ALL free glutamic acid contained in processed food. Wherever free glutamic acid is found, it should be referred to as MSG in public information (as I will throughout this book). That is not the case in today's markets. "MSG" never seems to be identified on food labels other than when it is associated with the use of the ingredient monosodium glutamate.

There is a great deal of awareness of the potential adverse reactions from monosodium glutamate. After Chinese Restaurant Syndrome had been identified, documented, and the information widely published, a stigma was attached to the use of monosodium glutamate in foods and we saw the words "monosodium glutamate" disappear from food labels on store shelves.

Today, less products list monosodium glutamate as an ingredient. And the popular catch phases often seen on labels, "No MSG" or "No Added MSG", compound the confusion. How accurate that statement may be is anyone's guess without knowledge of the complete ingredient lists. Or better yet, an analysis of the free glutamic acid content of the product at the time of its packaging, or even after it has sat on the shelves for awhile. There may be "no monosodium glutamate" in the products you use, however, there **may be** hidden free glutamic acid (MSG).

Those who need to provide ingredient information on food labels do so under Federal guidelines. These guidelines, discussed in a later chapter, allow companies to include ingredients which contain free glutamic acid (MSG) without listing the more commonly used term "MSG" on the label anywhere. In fact, there is no provision in these guidelines to indicate that there is any free glutamic acid contained as an ingredient at all.

Those of us who have been told by our medical professionals to avoid monosodium glutamate can do this by reading labels, but how do we avoid the rest of the manufactured free glutamic acid? You need to know where to look for it, but where?

The objective in a game of hide and seek is to hide and not be found. In the game we call *MSG Hide and Seek*, that can be perilous to those of us who are "IT". Lack of objective public information and rampant consumer confusion keep most of us searching.

The manufactures of monosodium glutamate and other ingredients that contain manufactured free glutamic acid use this lack of information and confusion we all have about our sensitivities to their advantage. If we were looking for foods without "MSG" and saw a product labeled "No MSG", that would lull us into believing that the product is "safe" for us to eat. We'd buy it and use it. (I know I would, because I have!)

If we had a reaction, the first thing we would do is look for the words "monosodium glutamate" or acronym "MSG" on the label. If we didn't find it there, we would wonder if our reactions were from "food poisoning", allergic reaction, intolerance or some other malady. (I used to get "food poisoning" at least twice a month!)

By learning about the common sources of MSG you can master your sensitivities by understanding them.

I know, first hand. The story is my own and those were the words of my own doctor in the early 1990's when my quest for a MSG FREE lifestyle began.

My greatest challenge, initially, was that I was only looking for sources of monosodium glutamate in my diet, so my journey towards wellness had many false starts, failures and setbacks. I also didn't realize at the time how pervasive a problem I had with MSG or how dramatically it effected so many areas of my life.

To make matters worse, there is a high degree of skepticism in the medical industry as to the affects of MSG in humans and a whole host of conflicting views. No one seemed to know what I suffered from, how to identify a path to wellness or even how to control my adverse reactions. I decided to strike out on my own and find some answers and finally to share them with others like you.

In a nutshell ...

The most important part of controlling your MSG sensitivities is to understand that it is dose related (how much you consume and your tolerance level may determine the type of reaction you may have and how much you must consume to have that reaction). Each person will experience different degrees of both adverse reactions and subsequently will react differently to the elimination of MSG from their diets.

The benefits can be far reaching and one benefit may lead to others.

- *You may experience weight loss and be able to maintain ideal weight more easily so you may diet less.*

- *You may experience a lessening of headaches, chest pain, shortness of breath, anxiety and be able to eliminate other substances (like over the counter and prescription medications) in your life which sport their own set of side effects and problems.*

- *Your skin may clear of acne, hives, sores, dryness and regain its health and radiance.*

- *You may experience more vitality, energy and ability to concentrate and focus on task, increasing your well being and productivity.*

- *Best of all, you get control back of how you feel.*

The bad news is that MSG can dramatically affect you physically. It can damage cells and have long term negative effects upon your system.

The good news is that the sources of the offending MSG (free glutamic acid) can be eliminated from your diet without having to make huge sacrifices to variety or life style. You can enjoy better health!

> *"It's been almost thirty years since: the first publicized report of any adverse reaction to MSG, the studies that followed, the formation of glutamate associations and thirty years of controversy on a substance that should never have been allowed to be added to food in the first place. Thirty years of reports of adverse reactions...you would think someone would have taken action on this by now."*
>
> Excerpts from a letter on file at the FDA

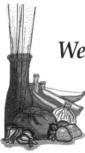

Welcome to "The Game"...

To understand how to play MSG Hide and Seek, it's best to get to know the players and the rules.

Let's start withthe players first.

Tag! You're IT!

Your body, wonder of the universe, is a complex web of materials that are interwoven into a complicated production system. When functioning at its peak, it is the envy of any modern manufacturing plant. Moment by moment, your biological system generates energy and byproducts to assist your body to breathe, pump blood, move, digest, think, feel and react.

It's all governed by a host of complex relationships based upon your genetic background, the amount of exercise you sustain, how you manage your mental state of mind and what you eat, drink and breath to fuel your system. Like any set of processes that make up a manufacturing system, your body will work only as smoothly as the sum of its total parts can function.

A key player in sustaining optimum health is your immune system. It is one of your greatest allies and yet can be your worst enemy. The immune system is responsible for fighting against infection, viruses, and other invading organisms. It has a marvelous set of tools that it can use to create an arsenal of weapons. One such weapon is the antibody. It can mount an immediate attack on the invader or store itself for later use.

It is when the immune system overreacts that it can become a hazard to its owner, causing allergic reactions and a whole host reactions they have to additives such as MSG as food allergies. That may not be the case. Let's look at why.

> "During my life I have suffered many adverse effects from ingesting manufactured free glutamic acid [MSG]...I had recurrent chest pain and tightness, an EKG revealed nothing... I passed out after lunch one day and the emergency room physician could find no explanation...another time my legs went numb, suspecting toxic shock I went to the emergency room, again, they could not explain it...[MSG] has severely interfered with my concentration abilities over the years, given me stomach cramps, has affected my vision and caused other problems [such as] migraine headaches...with much effort I sought out truthful information on MSG, reduced my intake of [MSG] and solved the migraine mystery."
>
> Excerpts from a letter on file at the FDA

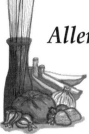

Allergies, Intolerance, and Chemical Sensitivities ...

It has been estimated that there are over 60 million Americans that suffer from allergies.

Allergies occur when the immune system suffers an abnormal overreaction to protein found in substances ingested, used topically or taken in by breathing. The immune system will bombard the foe with a frontal attack with the antibodies created to destroy it. This will often result in the host (the one that is experiencing the allergic reaction) suffering from runny nose, itchy eyes, swelling and other reactions.

Allergies differ greatly from intolerance or chemical sensitivities. Though they can be inter-related, as a person can simultaneously be allergic and or intolerant and or chemically sensitive. The differences in diagnosing any of these is that allergies can be confirmed fairly rapidly through the use of accepted procedures. Intolerance and sensitivities can only be determined through elimination and reintroduction of the suspected substance followed by close observation in controlled environments over extended periods of time.

Reactions, whether allergic, intolerant or chemically sensitive in nature, can happen within minutes, hours or days of exposure. That is why it is sometimes hard to pin down sensitivities to food and environmental substances. Most Americans vary their diets daily. The time lag between eating something and seeing a reaction may be too far apart to associate one with the other.

The methods of determining chemical sensitivities and intolerance for food are the same. A daily diary of exposure and reactions, along with the participation in an elimination diet is the recommended practice.

Allergies ...

The highest percentages of reactions caused by known allergens are attributed to pollen, dust, and mites, which all contain some protein.

What occurs is that the first time an allergen is introduced into the human body the immune system treats it as an enemy. The immune system begins to produce antibodies to defend itself against the invader and catalogs it in its memory. The next time the enemy is introduced into the system, the immune system kicks in and begins to release large amounts of histamines and other chemicals to combat the foe.

This overabundance of histamines and other substances can show up as a mild case of runny nose and sneezing to something as serious as anaphylactic shock and death. An overabundance of histamines in the system can also be uncomfortable in other ways. Symptoms including facial flushing, rash, vomiting, diarrhea and headaches are all associated with histamine intoxication; a form of food poisoning a histamine intolerant person may suffer.

There are several methods to test for allergic reactions to substances in your diet and lifestyle. There are many known reactions to foods such as peanuts, alfalfa, wheat, etc. An informed allergist is always the best source for current information on reactions and treatments.

One of the forms of testing is a scratch test. The patient has a small scratch or prick made on their skin (forearm or back) and a small amount of a suspected substance would be applied to the area. The area is monitored for reactions such as reddening, irritation, welting or itching. Reactions to pollen, vegetation, and animal dander are all diagnosed in this manner.

Another form is a RAST test in which blood is drawn from the patient and tested using potentially suspect substances. Amounts of the drawn blood and suspect materials are combined and studied for reactions.

Sometimes, allergies can only be pinpointed with daily diaries of use and reactions. Keeping a daily tally of what you eat and what adverse symptoms developed will help you in determining a pattern to any food allergies you may have. You can then eliminate the offending food for awhile and reintroduce it a week or two later. If you find that you react, you may have identified the offending food and you can eliminate it from your diet.

For some, the only way to make a positive identification of offending substances is to participate in an elimination diet. A strict diet of neutral food items is followed and other food items are introduced to challenge the patient's system into a reaction. A bit like Russian Roulette, it nevertheless is an effective method of identifying suspect allergens.

Intolerance ...

A good example of intolerance is in the inability of some people to digest milk products that contain lactose. When you are lactose intolerant, you lack the enzyme lactase in your system to properly digest and assimilate the enzyme.

If you are lactose intolerant, you might experience gas, bloating, and abdominal discomfort, nausea, vomiting, or other reactions from the ingestion of milk. Lactose - free milk products would cause you no reaction at all.

If you were allergic to milk products, however, and were to have milk or the lactose free milk, you would have allergic reactions to both products. This would happen because you suffer from allergies to the actual milk in both products.

Other types of intolerance mimic allergic or chemical sensitivity reactions. Celiac disease, or gluten intolerance, is often shown by poor food digestion and absorption, stomach upsets, diarrhea, abdominal cramps, bloating, mouth sores and an increased susceptibility to infections. Methylzanthine toxicity (related to caffeine or theobromine intolerance) can often cause distressing migraine headaches, palpitations, panic and anxiety attacks and vomiting, while sulfite intolerance can cause severe asthma attacks or shortness of breath.

Chemical Sensitivities ...

A chemically sensitive person reacts to additives, such as MSG, aspartame (NutraSweet®), sulfite, sulfates, nitrates, petroleum base dyes, flavors and preservatives. If the chemically sensitive person were to ingest either the milk or lactose-free milk product and it were to have an offending substance in it they would react to that substance, not the milk product. The ingestion of an unadulterated milk or lactose-free milk product may cause no reaction at all, unless, of course, the chemically sensitive person was also either allergic or intolerant to the milk, too.

So, when you are "reacting", are you allergic, intolerant or chemically sensitive? It's often hard to tell the difference. The bottom line is what may be causing you discomfort.

How you go about determining that will be how you determine if you are indeed, allergic to the actual organic substance, intolerant to some part or all of it; or are having chemical sensitivity reactions to additives used to enhance the substance.

"I was one of those millions who suffer from depression. I spent many hours and much money (both of my own health plan's and my own) on therapists trying to cope with the effects of depression on my personal and professional life. Because of weekly debilitating bouts of depression, I was unable to work beyond a clerical capacity despite the fact I had a college degree.

In 1983, I learned about a possible link between depression and MSG. I began to chart my food consumption and episodes of depression, and found that my onset of depression was always precipitated by consumption of MSG. It took 5 days for the effects of MSG to disappear. I diligently removed sources of MSG from my diet, and my depression was gone within a few days. Within a few months my income doubled. Because I was able to follow through on tasks and think more clearly, I received a promotion.

While I was never hospitalized because of a reaction to MSG, I would estimate the cost to me as follows:

Psychiatric, psychological and therapy sessions:	*$12,000*
Medical care [for related ills]:	*$15,000*
Lost wages due to Under-employment:(72-83)	*$111,000*
Lost wages due to restrictions on professional capability (83-97):	*unknown*

...I view my reaction to MSG as a disability. Like any disabled person, I can lead a productive and happy life if given the opportunity."

Excerpts from a letter on file at the FDA

So Who Gets To Play MSG Hide & Seek?

I personally believe that everyone reacts to MSG sooner or later. Regardless of your biological background, physical condition, weight, height, or sex, you can eventually consume enough MSG to cause yourself some problems.

After finding out that the root to most of my problems stemmed from MSG sensitivity, I began to ask others what "ills" seem to befall them regularly if the had mentioned they too felt they were MSG sensitive.

Responses of the types and severity of reactions vary wildly, though there are a few which most all of us suffer. The most common are "headaches" or more commonly referred to as "migraine headaches"; heart palpitations, shortness of breath and an incurable thirst.

Being aware of the side effects can help you to more clearly recognize when you ARE having a reaction and you can take steps to help yourself. Unfortunately, the "side effects" are so varied, it takes a "map" to figure it out. (See Page 38 for a listing of common reactions.)

Many people just live with the inconveniences, unaware that there is anything that could be done to alleviate their pain and distress. Most of you are left either undiagnosed or MIS-diagnosed due to a lack of understanding in the medical community of the host of ill effects one can suffer from excitotoxins like MSG in your diet. I contend that you don't have to suffer any longer, if MSG sensitivity is the root of your concerns, you can eliminate it from your life.

By following a few simple steps in modifying the foods and methods you use to prepare meals, you can identify offending substances in your diet. By eliminating them, you can see significant results.

"I'm a single working parent on a budget and have lost many days work...for many years, I've suffered with terrible headaches...triggered by then unknown sources...I've often thought I must be weak, that my pain and necessary life style changes that resulted [were] my fault, that I must be inferior in some way ...later I realized that I suffered from "classic migraines". These episodes are [the] direct result of different things that trigger them ...[such as] MSG, an additive I used in cooking to enhance flavor ... I consider myself fortunate as I know what [MSG] does to me but what about those Americans suffering other less dramatic effects: always thinking they're "slow" while their mother is busy in the kitchen cooking up something tasty with MSG."

Excerpts from a letter on file at the FDA

NOTE: Many health practitioners claim that certain amino acids, when taken as supplements, can help benefit your health overall. Though it is interesting to note that recently the FDA has considered reclassifying amino acid supplements as medicines; available by prescription only due to the abuse and subsequent adverse reactions of some to over the counter remedies such as tyrptophan used as a sleep aide.

Meet the Other Players of MSG Hide and Seek ...

MSG, Free Glutamic Acid, Monosodium Glutamate, and Hydrolyzed Proteins

MSG

It's probably best to begin this section with a clear understanding of the terms and terminology used in both industry and consumer circles when discussing MSG.

MSG sensitive consumers refer to what makes them ill as "MSG". What really causes their discomfort is either free glutamic acid that occurs in food 1) as a consequence of manufacture or 2) as a consequence of processing of proteins contained in food substances.

The ingredient monosodium glutamate is an ingredient that is 78% free glutamic acid. In the past, the acronym "MSG" was associated with only monosodium glutamate before consumers realized that ingredients other than monosodium glutamate were causing their MSG reactions. Today, the acronym is used as a phrase and "MSG" is used commonly by consumers to refer to any processed free glutamic acid found in food which causes MSG-like reactions.

What is MSG, really?
MSG has often been used as a flavor enhancer. It stimulates the taste buds and causes a person to experience a sensation of enhanced taste. When MSG is used in this way, its "job" is to enhance the taste of the food.

MSG can do this because it is a neurotransmitter. Neurotransmitters can transfer chemical information throughout the brain, carrying important information to different parts of the body. Neurotransmitters can cause neurons to fire. MSG creates a bigger taste by stimulating the neurons in the MSG receptive taste bud cells, causing them to "fire" rapidly, simulating an enhanced flavor. MSG can also be called a neurotoxin because it may make neurons fire repeatedly until they die of exhaustion.

Free Glutamic Acid ...

All protein is made up of complex strings of amino acids. Glutamic acid is an amino acid. When glutamic acid is found in protein it is referred to as "bound" glutamic acid. Bound glutamic acid found in human tissue is made of L-glutamic acid only.

When glutamic acid is freed from protein during digestion, the free glutamic acid is made up of L-glutamic acid only. No adverse reactions to the consumption of "protein", per sé, have been reported. But when glutamic acid is freed from protein due to processing before it is ingested, the glutamic acid changes significantly. The processing not only changes the glutamic acid it also creates byproducts-some of which have been found to be carcinogenic. (see Page 34 "Why glutamic acid may effect you?"). Also, any glutamic acid that has already been freed before you eat it doesn't have to be digested like the whole protein has to be digested. So instead of being released from the protein slowly, you can be exposed to a lot of processed free glutamic acid in a short period of time. Perhaps, at some point, too much for your system to handle and adverse reactions are the result.

L-glutamic acid is essential for normal body function. Humans do not need to eat protein in order to supply the body with the L-glutamic acid that it needs. If there is not enough L-glutamic acid available for normal body function, it can be created from other amino acids.

Amino acids, like glutamic acid, are critical components to the overall function of your biological system. There are tens of thousands of combinations of approximately 20 different amino acids, each combining in varying amounts to produce different types of proteins.

In reviewing over the counter or processed amino acid supplements, it is extremely important to note that to produce a supplement or additive one needs to process a great deal of raw materials to reduce it down to its purest form. This reduction is then again processed or combined with ingredients to allow it to be deliverable to the system, our bodies, in liquid, tablet, crystalline, salt or capsule form. This method is used to produce all supplements, even "natural" or "organically" derived.*

Monosodium Glutamate ...

Monosodium glutamate is an ingredient used in food. It is approximately 78% pure free glutamic acid (MSG). It is a food additive and excitotoxin. Monosodium glutamate is now generally manufactured by a fermentation process using bacteria and corn and is widely available at the grocer's in the form of a crystal similar to the appearance of salt or sugar. There is a greater concentration of MSG in the ingredient monosodium glutamate than in any other MSG- containing ingredient available.

Hydrolyzed Proteins
(Other Ingredients Containing MSG) ...

The FDA has essentially set up two groups of products containing MSG. One group is made up of glutamic acid and sodium that they call "monosodium glutamate" and a second group is made up of glutamic acid plus other chemicals and these ingredients are called hydrolyzed protein products. These products are often manufactured by a form of protein hydrolysis wherein the original substance is "broken down" by extreme or prolong exposure to high temperatures and/or an acid.

Another method is the use of enzymes to break down the protein during processing prior to ingestion. Many cheeses and other dairy products are produced in this way. Enzymes, which occur naturally in all foods, play an important role in our health. Using enzymes to predigest proteins, however, may result in additional byproducts that can negatively affect you.

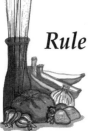

Rule One:
There are no clear rules ...

So, you're "IT", and we've met some of the players; MSG, free glutamic acid, monosodium glutamate and other MSG containing products called hydrolyzed proteins.

Now let's discuss the rules we use to play *MSG Hide and Seek*.

The Food and Drug Administration (FDA) has made up one of the key rules for our game of *MSG Hide and Seek*. This is specifically why we put special emphasis on your knowing about *hidden* sources of MSG.

Their ruling goes something like this:

> *When a product is approximately 78% pure MSG (free glutamic acid) and salt, the product is called "monosodium glutamate" by the FDA and must be labeled as such. However, when a hydrolyzed protein contains less than 78% MSG (free glutamic acid) in combination with salt, the FDA does not require that the words "monosodium glutamate", "glutamate", or phrase "MSG" appear on a product's label as part of the ingredient listings.*

"Autolyzed yeast", "hydrolyzed soy protein" and "sodium caseinate" are examples of names given to hydrolyzed proteins used for ingredients on food labels that contain high levels of MSG.

To add to the confusion, the "Glutamate Industry", those that manufacture monosodium glutamate and hydrolyzed protein products, and the FDA, use the phrase "MSG" as an acronym for the ingredient called monosodium glutamate. If a consumer were to ask, "Is there any MSG in your product," they would be told "No" unless the product contains the ingredient monosodium glutamate.

Both monosodium glutamate and hydrolyzed proteins can be used interchangeably as flavor enhancers in foods. As I have stated before, both contain free glutamic acid (MSG). From my point of view, they belong in the same category, governed by the same rules.

Manufacturers can use hydrolyzed protein products at will without notification of their contribution of free glutamic acid (MSG) content in the products you buy. It isn't unusual to have multiple sources of free glutamic acid (MSG) in the form of the above ingredients, along with many others, in any given processed food. (see chart Page 44)
Food items need not be labeled as containing "MSG" in any way. Only if there is use of monosodium glutamate will there ever be a clue to the consumer as to the presence of MSG.

My advice is to refer to Rule One.

How is it used?

Asians have used seaweed as a flavor enhancer for at least 2,000 years in the form of a broth made with a type of seaweed known as sea tangle. Boiling the seaweed breaks down its proteins and releases free glutamic acid. In order

NOTE: There are many theories as to how MSG works to enhance flavors. It may increase the sensitivity of the taste buds; it may increase salivation, which may increase the perception of flavor. It has also been suggested that MSG stimulates the receptors in the mouth and tongue *"creating sensations like no spice can"*.

to justify its use, the Glutamate Industry promotes MSG as a fifth taste, past salty, sweet, sour, or bitter and it is a common base or addition to most recipes. I find monosodium glutamate to make foods taste "tinny" and with any type of MSG, the immediate dryness in my mouth helps me identify foods that contain it, though I can't personally identify a specific taste, only sensation.

In the US Market, free forms of glutamic acid can be found in food, cosmetics and medications. Studies completed on its use here in 1995 show that the food industry leads market usage; restaurants and institutions (schools, hospitals, nursing homes, etc) use the most followed closely by convenience food distribution channels (prepared and packaged foods). Next were packaged soups, seasoning blends and then bottled monosodium glutamate packaged and sold as salts or crystals.

MSG is not like a spice such as salt, oregano or pepper. These lend their own taste to food. Free glutamic acid essentially has no taste of its own. It's core strength is its ability to stimulate receptors in your brain, telling your senses, much like a drug, that what you are tasting is a larger, more robust taste than the food itself might portray on its own.

A market is born...

The Asian industry saw the potential commercial value of the food additive monosodium glutamate shortly after the turn of the century. It reached the United States, in quantity, shortly after World War II. By mid 1960, production reached over 40 million pounds per year here in America. A recent report on worldwide usage projected that monosodium glutamate had a total world market capacity of over 1,100 thousand metric tons. Monosodium glutamate and, more recently, hydrolyzed vegetable proteins and other forms of free glutamic acid are sold in both consumer packaging (available by the bottle) and as a commodity to food purveyors for use in commercial food preparation.

The top 3 producers of MSG are Ajinomoto Co., Inc. (Japan), Tung Hai Fermentation Industrial Corp. (Taiwan) and Miwon Co., Ltd. (Rep of Korea). Most manufacture of MSG is centered in the Pacific Rim. There are plants in 15 countries in the world including the United States, Brazil, Peru, and France. Interestingly, the US imports billions of dollars of MSG and monosodium glutamate. The lion's share is received from Asia and South America.

There is only one manufacturing plant currently left operating here in the United States (Archer Daniels Midland in North Carolina). It was recently stated that they will cease operations after fulfilling orders through 1998 and close up shop. A multi-billion dollar US market of a product that is mostly made from corn and we have no plants within our own shores?

How does it work?

The common usage of MSG required it to be defined. As there was no adequate description to use, those involved with food science (biochemical engineering) came up with a new term; "potentiator". In pharmacology, the term potentiation is the "action of an agent" enhancing the effects of other agents upon a system.

If you look at your body as a biological system, it makes sense to define MSG and its effects as a potentiator. Again, the potentiator does not contribute any taste by itself but merely stimulates the system into thinking that it does.

Another term used for MSG is "excitotoxin"; a phrase neuroscientists coined to describe chemicals such as free glutamic acid, L-cysteine and aspartic acid (in aspartame-NutraSweet®) which excite and kill cells in the nervous system. Excitotoxins over stimulate the neurons making them fire repeatedly which can lead to cell exhaustion and cell death.

The connection between these excitotoxins and obesity, reproductive challenges, physical growth and neurodegenerative diseases (such as Parkinson's, Alzheimer's, Huntington's and others) is alarming. Dr. John Olney, MD, a neuroscientist, and others showed a direct effect of excitotoxins to damage nerve cells in the brain and retina. (Medical journal references are listed in the Appendix F.)

For more information, review a copy of "*In Bad Taste. The MSG Syndrome*" by George R. Schwartz, M.D., It was written in 1990 and discusses the work of Olney and others. Or a recently released book written by Dr. Russell Blaylock; "*Excitotoxins, The Taste that Kills*" (1997). Both gentleman are published and recognized doctors; Schwartz being an internationally recognized physician and toxicologist and Blaylock a practicing board-certified neurosurgeon with a deep understanding of neurodegenerative diseases. Their work shows the potential damage excitotoxins such as MSG (free glutamic acid), aspartic acid and L-cysteine can cause to the human condition. It is overwhelming.

Conditions such as mitral valve prolapse (MVP), asthma, chronic fatigue syndrome (CFS, CFIDS), migraine headaches, behavioral disorders like attention deficit disorder and attention deficit hyperactive disorder (ADD, ADHD), violent behavior, bed wetting, sleep disorders and heart problems may all have ties to MSG sensitivity and the use of excitotoxins in your diet. MSG may trigger these conditions, simply worsen them or confuse the effect and subsequent diagnosis and treatment.

We simply have not spent the time and money to discover why MSG and other excitotoxins cause adverse reactions. Little or no independent funding is available to study these issues outside the monosodium glutamate industry itself. In the US, we leave the bulk of the responsibility of research and product safety testing for products like breast implants, drugs and tobacco to the manufacturers to prove their products safety. "Independent" testing and study often dismiss any correlation between use of MSG and ailments that would adversely effect the manufacturing community or impact the large import that MSG brings to our economy.

It is very hard to regulate a multi-billion dollar international industry, so finding and following your own self help program is one of the best paths towards your success.

Why Might Free Glutamic Acid Affect You?
It is very important to understand the difference between glutamic acid freed from protein during digestion and the free glutamic acid that is created by a manufacturing process. To go through this information requires some technical detail, but I'll work at keeping it simple.

Glutamic acid, found in higher organisms, only contains L-glutamic acid and nothing more. When free glutamic acid is created prior to ingestion, by hydrolyzation, fermentation or use of enzymes (enzymolysis) a mirror image of the L-glutamic acid is actually created. It is referred to as

D-glutamic acid. The amount of free glutamic acid created is dependent on the source of the protein used and the extent of the hydrolysis, fermentation or enzymolysis.

Along with this shift in its make up, the manufacture of free glutamic acid causes a variety of chemical reactions and a range of unwanted byproducts. Manufactured free glutamic acid is made up of L-glutamic acid and D-glutamic acid and may bring with it pyroglutamic acid, mono & dichloro propanols (MCP & DCP) and heterocyclic amines. The propanols and heterocyclic amines are all carcinogenic.

The glutamic acid found in our bodies and in uncooked, unadulterated food proteins (tomatoes, mushrooms, peas, etc) contains only L-glutamic acid. D-glutamic acid is not found in higher organisms, though it can be found in the walls of some bacteria. It has not been concluded whether differences between D-glutamic acid and L-glutamic acid are what causes sensitivity; but it is clear that only D-glutamic acid seems to cause MSG sensitive people adverse reactions.

When protein is eaten, chains of amino acids are broken apart slowly during the digestive process. It is believed that when MSG itself is ingested a rapid assimilation of MSG occurs bringing it into the blood stream, raising the normal amount of glutamic acid in the blood to eight to ten times the normal amount. The mechanism may be much more complex than simple elevated blood levels. Researchers have recently found large concentrations of MSG outside of the blood stream, in cerebo-spinal fluid. We have a lot to learn about MSG reactions.

Studies have shown that L-glutamic acid is used in our brains as a nerve impulse transmitter (neurotransmitter) and that there are glutamate-responsive tissues in other parts of the

NOTE: It is estimated that 30% of us suffer adverse reactions from the ingestion of MSG in a normal diet.

body as well. Abnormal function of glutamate receptors has been linked with certain neurological diseases such as Alzheimer's, Amyotrophic Lateral Sclerosis (ALS), Parkinson and Huntington's disease. Ingestion of MSG may exacerbate these conditions.

A report published in 1995 from the Federation of American Societies for Experimental Biology (FASEB) identified two groups that are particularly at risk ingesting MSG; those who may be intolerant to MSG: when MSG is consumed "in a large quantity" and those that have severe, poorly controlled asthma. The report concluded that it took only .5 (1/2) gram (approximately 1/10th of a teaspoonful) to provoke adverse reactions in some people.

As implied by the report from FASEB, sensitivity to free glutamic acid is dose related. Considering the grand amount of potential sources of free glutamic acid in the average American diet, it is no wonder that our systems may become overburdened and start reacting. Your genetic background, associated allergies and intolerance, height, weight, and general state of good health may all contribute to your sensitivity to MSG.

Read the labels of foods in your cupboards. Check with your local restaurant haunts and begin to consider how much free glutamic acid you may be ingesting in the foods you eat, in each meal; daily; weekly. The summary report given by FASEB would have us believe that approximately 3 grams a day (slightly less than a teaspoonful) was a reasonable amount to ingest with little or no side effects or sensitivity reactions to "most people". But, individual studies cited in the FASEB report give examples of reactions to .5 (1/2) grams of MSG.

Unfortunately, no study has ever been done to determine how small of an amount of MSG could trigger a reaction.

It is only the processed free glutamic acid that appears to cause MSG sensitive individuals problems. That is why understanding where you will find processed free glutamic acid is critical. Not only are there ingredients that contain free glutamic acid intentionally (see chart Page 44), but, also, there are products that contain proteins which may create MSG during manufacture or after packaging. Certain forms of yeast or enzymes combined with protein manufacture MSG. Often, the mere aging of one of these products may cause additional amounts of free glutamic acid to develop.

Some of the foods that might be suspect are cheese, low fat dairy products, yogurt, fermented or hydrolyzed items such as vinegar, yeast, tofu and soy products. All may cause adverse reactions to the MSG sensitive person, even if they come from organic sources. Fresh, uncooked, organically grown produce such as tomatoes and mushrooms, which contain glutamic acid, do not seem to cause these severe reactions in MSG sensitive people. Again, this may be because these foods contain L-glutamic acid and NO D-glutamic acid.

Tip #1: Optimum Menu Planning ...

Any item that contains protein will contain glutamic acid and any processed food may contain some amount of free glutamic acid. Keep this in mind as you plan your menus. Glutamic acid bound up in protein when you eat it is of no consequence (such as steak, eggs, fish). However, if the item's protein is hydrolyzed (heated to extreme temperatures, or cooked overly well), fermented (including over ripening), or treated with enzymes (most processed cheeses, sour creams, low and skim dairy products) the item is suspect of being able to cause adverse reactions.

MSG Reactions:
Common Adverse Reported Reactions

Cardiac
Angina
Arrhythmias
Extreme drop in blood
  pressure
Numbness or paralysis
Rapid heartbeat
  (tachycardia)
Seizures
Slurred speech

Circulatory
Swelling

Digestive
Bloating
Diarrhea
Irritable bowel
Nausea/vomiting
Stomach cramps

Muscular
Flu-like achiness
Joint pain
Stiffness

Neurological
Anxiety
Depression
Disorientation
Dizziness
Light-headedness
Loss of balance
Mental confusion
Panic attacks

Neurological (con't)
Behavioral problems
  (ADD/ADHD)
Drowsiness
Hyperactivity
Insomnia
Lethargy
Migraine headache

Respiratory
Asthma
Shortness of breath
Chest pain
Tightness
Runny nose
Sneezing

Skin
Extreme dryness of the
  mouth
Flushing
Hives or rash
Mouth lesions
Temporary tightness or
  partial paralysis
  (numbness or tingling)
  of the skin

Urological
Nocturia (bed wetting)
Swelling of prostate
Prostrate Abnormalities

Visual
Blurred vision
Difficulty focusing

Information courtesy of the *Truth in Labeling Campaign.*

The amount of the processed free glutamic acid that you consume is the important factor to consider in choosing a diet that will help you obtain optimum health. The conversation is about dosage. Regardless of the form you ingest it in, sooner or later, you will probably consume enough to cause yourself a reaction.

Tip #2: Common Reactions ...

Millions of people worldwide show signs of MSG sensitivity with reactions ranging from mild to very severe. The most common symptoms generally reported after a chemical sensitivity reaction to food or ingredients is migraine headaches. Reported physical symptoms related to MSG sensitivity are: heartburn, diarrhea, abdominal cramps, unusual thirst, seizures, asthma, nausea, burning, tightness, numbness in the upper chest, neck and face, tingling, warmth, a feeling of pressure about the head or headache, heart palpitations, chest pain, ear ringing, depression, sleeplessness, drowsiness; a whole host of side effects (see Chart Page 38).

MSG reactions can mock the most dramatic allergic reaction, intolerance or neurological drug side effect that you can name. People have been diagnosed as having such maladies as mitral valve prolapse, ADD/ADHD, asthma, brain lesions, neurosis, functional colitis and depression, when in fact their illness may have been brought on or exacerbated by MSG.

Medical practitioners familiar with MSG sensitivity, have used MSG to challenge patients with the above conditions. ("Challenging" them by eliminating the substance for a short time and then reintroducing it back into their diets or challenging them in their offices.) The resulting reactions, simulating the symptoms, promote the reevaluation of their diagnosis and after diet modification, their patients have shown significant improvement.

The most important discovery that has been made in my opinion is that MSG reactions are dose related. What may affect one may not affect another. I can't tolerate much more than what might be contained on one seasoned chip or cracker before experiencing reactions. My immediate reactions are a dry sensation in my mouth, thirst and a headache. More interestingly, hours or even days later, I may also suffer from abdominal cramping, gas, diarrhea other symptoms such as depression, after eating a painfully small amount.

More than a few grams at once and you will find me in the restroom, violently ill within 15 minutes to an hour.

The most interesting phenomena that I have noted about my MSG reaction is the seemingly unrelated emotional and psychological reactions I experience. Mood swings, lack of emotional control, added stress and anxiety are all common for me after eating MSG, in any quantity. It has been noted repeatedly that reactions to MSG vary greatly from individual to individual. No wonder our medical community seems to have a hard time determining what might be effecting those of us with MSG reactions. Identifying your sensitivities to MSG may well be your first step towards wellness if you are challenged by these

NOTE: No one knows whether MSG causes the condition underlying the reaction or whether the underlying condition is simply aggravated by the ingestion of MSG. We only know that the reactions listed on page 38 are sometimes caused or exacerbated by ingestion of MSG. All forms of MSG (free glutamic acid that occurs in food as a consequence of manufacture or processing) cause these reactions in MSG-sensitive people. As a side note, the ingestion of alcohol and other drugs, along with MSG, is suspected to enhance its adverse reactions.

or other problems. Always check with your medical practitioner before making any changes to your current diet or medication schedules.

If your medical practitioner is unfamiliar with current studies in this area, there are some reading sources in Appendix F for their review.

How can I tell if I am sensitive to MSG?

Unfortunately there is no test for MSG sensitivity; no blood work, brain scan or skin test available that will determine if you are truly "MSG-sensitive". Complicating matters is that there are many other suspect products that you may also be sensitive to as well. (See Appendices D & E) The only "test" that can help you to truly determine the source of your symptoms is called a "challenge".

"Challenge" is a term used in the medical industry to define a type of testing process in which the potential culprit must be first removed from use and then reintroduced under "a truth or dare" scenario. The "patient" (we will call them for our purposes here) is asked to remove the offending product(s) from their lifestyle. Then the patient is given the potentially reactive substance and observed.

Remember that there is more than one place for MSG to hide. When a protease enzyme or other reactive agent is allowed to interact with protein during product manufacture MSG is produced. This can bring on these same adverse reactions in MSG sensitive persons as intentionally added ingredients like hydrolyzed protein.

There is often no clue on the product label that such an interaction is taking place. Somewhat of a clue is to look for the presence of a dairy ingredient (like cheese) along with "protease enzymes" or "enzymes" added.

As an example, I had purchased and consumed a snack food item with the following ingredients and suffered as dramatic a reaction as I would have ingesting monosodium glutamate. The product ingredients were yellow cornmeal, expeller pressed hi-oleic canola oil, aged cheddar and blue cheese (milkfat, nonfat dry milk, salt, cheese cultures, enzymes), whey, buttermilk solids, sea salt, lactic acid, spices (paprika, annatto, turmeric).

About 45 minutes after we snacked on these during a ride home, I thought I was going to die. My face and neck were flushed and I had an extreme thirst and headache. My abdomen was extended with gas and I had to rush to the restroom with diarrhea. Well into the next day, I suffered from joint and muscle pain and dizziness. Of course, feeling like this did nothing for my temperament, and I was moody and distant until the symptoms passed.

No hint that any of these ingredients contained MSG was indicated on the label yet I suffered the consequences as if I had monosodium glutamate. The cornmeal, aged cheddar and blue cheeses, whey and buttermilk solids probably contained free glutamic acid (MSG) and caused my severe reactions. So much for simply avoiding "MSG"; now you see why we call the game *MSG Hide and Seek*.

Tip #3: Common Sources of MSG

There is evidence of MSG in almost every product category on the market today - foods, medicines, and cosmetics. You, by way of food combining and preparing food can manufacture MSG in your own kitchen. Aging processes and additives used in "enriched" products (breads, flour, and pasta) will all add MSG to the product.

By eliminating sources of MSG that are commercially available, you can begin to experience the benefits of a lower level of MSG in your system right away. After that, you can hone in on the other sources or causes of MSG reactions in your diet and lifestyle and eliminate them too.

Learn the sources of MSG. The following chart (Page 44) is a list of *hidden* sources of MSG. Feel free to copy and distribute this list with our permission. To be kept informed on a more regular basis, contact Truth in Labeling Campaign who supplied the original information. (Their contact information is in Appendix C.)

This list is compiled from sources of MSG that are available in today's market. Production and the sale of hydrolyzed proteins and autolyzed yeast products are basically unregulated. New names for the same MSG will, no doubt, creep into our distribution cycles as time goes by. In the event that the FDA approves the common use of irradiation on commercially available foods, there may be more *hidden* sources of MSG in the future.

Common Names and Phrases Often Used for Ingredients that Contain or Create MSG

Autolyzed yeast
Barley malt
Bouillon
Broth
Calcium caseinate
Carmel flavoring
Carrageenan
Enriched and protein
   fortified products
"Food Starch" of any kind
   (Wheat, Potato, etc)
Flavor(s)
Flavorings(s)
Free glutamic acid
Fungal protease
Gelatin
Guar gum
Hydrolyzed protein
Hydrolyzed vegetable
   protein
Protease
Protease enzymes
Malted barley
Malt extract
Malt flavoring
Maltodextrin
Modified food starch

Modified corn starch
Modified potato starch
Monosodium glutamate
   glutamate
Monopotassium
   glutamate
Natural flavor(s)
Natural pork, chicken and
   beef flavoring(s)
Pectin
Seasonings
Sodium caseinate
Soy sauce
Soy protein
Soy extract
Soy protein isolates
Soy protein concentrate
Smoke flavoring
Stock
Textured proteins
Whey protein
Whey protein isolates
Whey protein concentrate
Yeast extract
Yeast food
Yeast nutrient
Xanthum gum

Information courtesy of the *Truth in Labeling Campaign*.

Check with your pharmacist, too. Binders and fillers for medications, nutrients, and supplements, both prescription and non-prescription, including enteral feeding materials and some fluids administered intravenously in hospitals, may contain free glutamic acid. Maltodextrin, gelatin, cornstarch and other products that may contain MSG are commonly used in tablets and capsules. Injected medication may contain preservatives, that you may react to even if they do not contain MSG.

Cough medications (child and adult types) contain various suspect items such as corn syrup, flavorings and a host of items on the MSG *Hidden Sources* lists. Approximately 40% of children's over the counter medications contain aspartame (a known excitotoxin).

MSG and Your Child's Food

I had an enlightening experience in doing research for this book. I set about one day to "catalog the grocery store" of all the foods that you might find that you could eat with some comfort if you were MSG sensitive. I found myself in the infant food section and became fascinated at what I found there.

I checked the sections for newborn through toddler foods. What might be called "stage one" jar foods for babies seemed to be quite void of any type of food additives. There were the standard brands and new ones that seemed to focus on delivering "organic" baby foods, too. I was relieved to find that there is sacred ground in packaged foods after all.

"Stage Two" foods showed little use of anything more suspect than "broth" with some of the meat items and added citric acid (which may be derived from corn) in some of the fruits. "Broth" is an ingredient with *hidden* meaning. How and what

create the "broth" isn't noted on the label. It is on
Sources list and could be suspect.

After "Stage Two", the labels read like the text of a chemical
digest. Various forms of free glutamic acid were in every jar or
packaged food I picked off the shelf. If fed exclusively from the
"jar", at the tender age of what, 12 to 18 months, our children
could be exposed to a whole host of MSG sources in every
meal. If I couldn't eat it with some confidence myself, I surely
wouldn't trust it to my child.

Use the *Hidden Sources* list to review the labels on toddler foods
and other "table food" you may feed your child. Review
Excitotoxins: The Taste that Kills, or any of a number of studies
listed in the Appendices. You will find information on studies
of the effects of MSG and other excitotoxins (like aspartame).
Studies have shown evidence of adverse effects from free
glutamic acid on the hypothalamus and the retina. It may have
life long effects on your child's vision, weight, growth, fertility,
attention span, general health and personality.

Meats/Fish/Poultry/Seafood

The United Stated Department of Agriculture (USDA) regulates
animal products and does not require labeling for meats and
poultry prepared or processed using hydrolyzed proteins.
Butcher wrapped meats don't have ingredient lists the last time
I checked. Your purest source of unprocessed and
unadulterated animal or fish protein is a trusted butcher or
meat counter in a local health food store that carries "natural"
or "organic" items. Organic foods, grown under the California
Organic Food Act cannot, by definition, contain antibiotics,
sulfates, nitrates, phosphates, steroids, toxins from feed,
pesticides and chemicals used in processing and preserving.
The Organic Food Act, does NOT, however, set any guidelines

for the use of hydrolyzed proteins or autolyzed ye.
marinades, soy products, packaged protein or tender.
products may all contain suspect hidden sources of MSG.

Dairy Products and MSG

It may be wise to avoid dairy foods as you explore your MSG
sensitivity. If you wish to include them, use only whole food
products (whole milk and butter) from organic sources and
check labels carefully to reduce your exposure to MSG.
Synthetic pesticides, herbicides, fertilizers and milk production
hormones like rBGH are all prohibited by organic certification.
Again, however, hydrolyzed protein products are not. Many
products (even ones that are labeled "all natural" or "organic")
such as cheese, sour cream, butter, low fat or skim dairy
products may contain MSG. Check their labels for carrageenan,
xanthum gum, modified food starch, enzymes, and protease
enzymes, etc.

Salts and Sugars

Any "boxed or packaged" products might contain MSG.
Enrichment, flowing agents and fillers may all contain MSG.
Powered sugars and baking powder may contain cornstarch.
Using organic sea salt and cane sugar may help you avoid
additives.

Fats/ Oils and Butters

It's common belief that a low fat diet is a healthy one.
Processed "low fat" products may often contain high amounts
of free glutamic acid due to their method of production.
Removal of fat reduces flavor. Free glutamic acid is added to
"boost" the flavor and make low fat foods palatable. Many of
these foods such as margarine are created by the use of
enzymes creating free glutamic acid from what little protein
was contained in the dairy they originate from.

. you do choose to use fats, oils or butter; use whole-unadulterated products; extra virgin olive oils and organic butters and fats.

Eggs

Undyed, organic range-free eggs are a great source of protein.

Phase One:
The Modified Elimination

I drained my pocket book before I decided to look at my diet for answers to my health problems. I went to every known type of medical source in my metro area in search of answers; cardiologists for my heart murmur and arrhythmia; general practitioners for colds, flu and other maladies; my OB/GYN for PMS; chiropractors for muscle and joint pains, osteopathic doctors (DO) and naturopaths for nutrition and lifestyle counseling.

What I found was that the representatives I saw from the western medical community seemed unknowledgeable and unsympathetic to my condition and its cause. Often, the issue of remedies was brought up, but they were always solutions that merely masked the symptoms. Never was my diet or lifestyle ever questioned. Desperate, I turned to the alternative medical community for help. That was not an instant success either! I was tested for parasites, fungal infections, viruses; all to no avail. A friend suggested I go to see someone who might know more about diet and nutrition. I saw a dietician recommended by my general practitioner. She asked a lot of great questions and came up with the same conclusion as my GP; stay away from monosodium glutamate, but offered no other information.

I eliminated all the *monosodium glutamate* from my diet. Everything, every last item. I still got sick. Not one person mentioned the relationship of *monosodium glutamate* to *free glutamic acid.*

I happened upon a naturopath that had recently opened his doors in my community. In his office, I picked up a book on cleansing your system by way of an elimination diet. We discussed the program and created a plan. I was to go through a serious adjustment to my eating habits to discover my cure. The naturopath provided the needed support and I set about to tame my tiger.

We were still missing some critical information for the first few weeks. What, besides monosodium glutamate, might be causing my problems continued to elude us. Just removing that didn't seem to affect much. We also needed to eliminate my potential food allergies and intolerance and then hone in on specific ingredients. We were at this for a couple of weeks and it seemed like we were getting nowhere.

During some library research, I happened upon a listing of NO MSG, an educational and support group. I contacted them and was amazed that 1) the volunteer manning the phone understood what I was talking about 2) identified with my problems personally and 3) could provide me with more information about MSG than any medical group I ever encountered had in the past. I immediately sent for a subscription to their newsletter and list of commons sources of MSG. With this list of *Hidden Sources*, we were now loaded for bear.

Why Should I Do an Elimination ...
The first step in helping to identify a challenging substance in a system is to reduce the components of the system to its simplest form. You can identify offending foods, medicines and cosmetic items in your life by taking them away for a short time and then slowly re-introducing them into your life.

An elimination diet is often the only method that can isolate offending substances such as food additives without a doubt. It is used by allergists, cardiologists, nutritionists and others to help identify and treat many afflictions. A full elimination diet can be extremely restrictive, and should be undertaken with a great deal of thought and with the assistance of a dietician, nutritionist or medical practitioner. The suggestions I make here are to avoid products containing suspect additives such as MSG and other chemical additives, which is why I call this a "modified" elimination.

The closer you follow the modified elimination the greater your potential of success.

I am a product of my generation; fast food; prepared meals; eating out is all a very common part of my life-style and diet. To succeed in correctly identifying what was affecting me - I needed to make the commitment to simplify my diet, evaluate what I ate and record any reaction for a few weeks. It wasn't easy at first - but it has been well worth the efforts.

Getting Started ...
The whole point of this modified elimination is to remove all the free glutamic acid (MSG) sources from your diet. You won't see a dramatic shift in the meals that you plan, though you will surely experience a shift in how you will shop for ingredients and how you prepare your meals. You can taper into the modified elimination, though results will be slower coming.

To insure your success, I hope to provide you some stepping stones towards positive results. By eliminating obvious sources of MSG in your diet, you should see marked results; however, to really see overall benefits you may need to consider making radical changes to your overall lifestyle. Consult a health professional before launching into any dramatic changes. Your first goal is to merely eliminate the free glutamic acid (MSG) in your diet.

The Basics ...

In my research, I found that there are some extremely restrictive elimination diets that medical experts can put you on to challenge you for food allergies and sensitivities. After you have worked through the "modified elimination" that I suggest, if you still find little or no results, you should see a medical practitioner, knowledgeable in this field, to discuss a more intense review of your situation.

For now, you are merely attempting to eliminate the chemical and artificial additives you have in your diet that you have grown complacent to eating. You probably don't need to make huge changes to your menu planning to see significant results, just keep some of these simple suggestions in mind as you shop and prepare food for yourself and your family.

Step one: Planning...

Take the time to create a meal plan, especially if you have never done this before. If you do, you can shop in advance for food items you may want on hand and it will help you eliminate substitutions that may fall outside what you wish to eat.

Plan for snacks to be included! I would recommend that you eat whenever you are hungry. Small portions of crackers, cut vegetables, hard boiled eggs, dried fruits, fruit leathers or unflavored popcorn can satisfy your need to crunch, munch or at worst, "cheat". Find something that is easily portable, so you can keep it with you.

I have crackers or popcorn around all the time to keep the "rumbles" away and pep me up when my energy gets low. I also like organic fruit leathers. My local health food store has them in self-wrapped packages and they are very easy to keep in my purse, car or office drawer for long periods of time. Keep an eye out for use of thickeners or pectin! If you have a dehydrator, homemade fruit leather made from clean, organic fruits is the best!

Step Two: Eat Healthy

It is very important to consume only the healthiest of foods. Obtain organic vegetables, dairy, meat, carbohydrate, starch and condiment products and prepare them with minimal spices and processing (cooking).

If you live in the city or if you are watching a budget, you might find purchasing organic vegetables, produce, meats and other products a hardship. In this event, always wash or peel conventionally grown vegetables and produce before you eat it. You should avoid "enriched" foods (bread, flours, and pasta) as they can contain a whole host of MSG laden ingredients. Ask your grocer about special orders!

Step Three: Simplify

Though you will want to eat foods from every main food group daily, there is no rule that says you must eat from each of these groups at every meal! One of the best ways to help digestion and food assimilation is to keep the number and types of foods that you eat in a single meal to a minimum. The menu suggestions on Page 55 are kept simple for that reason. If you follow this example, you will also be combining your foods for optimum digestibility.

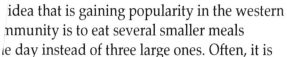

idea that is gaining popularity in the western nmunity is to eat several smaller meals ie day instead of three large ones. Often, it is suggested that these meals begin early in the morning with fruit and add vegetables, carbohydrates, and then complex carbohydrates, ending well before bedtime with heavier foods such as diary and proteins towards the end of the day.

For best digestion; eat fruit alone and early in the day; do not combine starches and proteins, or drink with meals. If you'd like some fluids, drink 15 minutes before a meal and wait for an hour after eating before consuming anything.

For more information on the benefits of proper food combining refer to books like *Fit for Life* by Harvey & Marilyn Diamond or the *New Book of Food Combining* by Jan Dries, listed in the book section of the Appendices. There are super recipes and great tips in each book. Avoid the recipes with ingredients from the *Hidden Sources* list and foods such as corn, cornstarch and dairy for the first few weeks of your elimination. Add them back into your diet slowly, one at a time.

Prepare your own food until you know that you have your sensitivities well identified and under control.

If you are allergic to or intolerant of known foods, avoid them as you would normally.

The following is a suggestion for you to use to do meal planning around, nothing more. While on this modified elimination, we are not counting calories. As soon as you normalize and reduce your body's intake of MSG, you may see a dramatic shift in your weight as a result anyway.

Sample Meal Plan

* **Breakfast:** *have only fresh fruit and fresh fruit juices from concentrates or those with added citric acid (A Hidden Sources list item).*

* **Mid-morning:** *enjoy heavier fresh fruits such as apples or bananas; fruit chips from your dehydrator or snack on crackers and butter. Butters are pretty neutral, though I have found specific brand that I like to use best (check "Annie's Cupboard" list).*

   Don't mix fruit with your starch or eat starch products with fruit in them (even if you made them). Fruits and other foods digest differently and can create additional gas and digestive challenges. These are discomforts we are trying to minimalize!

   If the muffin came from a package, the processing of the fruit may have added sulfite, corn syrup, dextrose or other items that are so minimal that they may not appear on the packaging. Err on the side of your success and leave them for later!

* **Lunch:** *have a vegetable salad or veggie sandwich, rice or potatoes and vegetables, or a protein and vegetables.*

   Eat vegetables cleaned and raw or steam them lightly in pure water only. A bit of sea salt, herbs and unadulterated whole butter is a great added touch.

   Lemon juice is a great substitute for vinegar in salads. Use pure virgin olive oils, herbs, sea salt and pure peppers to liven up the taste. One of my favorite salads is a squeeze of lemon, tablespoon of olive oil and fresh chopped basil, dash of sea salt, pepper with a pinch of dill tossed with sprouts and chopped tomatoes, cucumbers and red or yellow bell pepper

* **Mid-Day**: *have a snack of crackers, chips or nuts*

* **Supper (early evening)**: *unenriched pasta, potatoes or brown rice and vegetables or protein and vegetables; or dairy and vegetables*

* **Dinner (late evening, 3-4 hours before bed)**: *unenriched pasta, potatoes, brown rice and steamed vegetables or a starchy snack*

> *For the first couple of weeks, you might want to avoid animal protein from conventional sources. They are suspect to additives that may cause you reactions (especially poultry and seafood) and don't even think of eating luncheon meats, hot dogs or other packaged meats. They contain high levels of sulfite, salts and often are treated with corn syrup, food starch, dextrose and colored with "caramel" which is derived from corn and molasses.*

Here's some starting tips...

• *Do the meal plan, at least at first. Take it to your local grocer and check on the availability of items you need.*

• *Go through your cupboards and refrigerator and put aside or throw away what ever is there that contains suspect ingredients.*

• *Avoid fresh seafood and fish the first few weeks as their handlers are not required to report on products used in processing such as phosphates and sulfite used to preserve them. Take the time to locate a good source for later!*

• *Avoid using prepared sauces and condiments, especially soy, during the first few weeks. Some soy products are fermented protein and can also have additional additives.*

• *Avoid mayonnaise made with eggs, animal oils and other preservatives or additives for the first few weeks of your modified elimination. There are a few alternatives to brands that we all grew up with in the health food stores. (I included a family recipe in the Appendices - See Appendix G)*

• *Commercially available ketchup and mustards, due to the processed ingredients also need to be either avoided or changed to organic brands with no preservatives, formaldehyde, citric acid, dextrose or other offending items. Sea salt, pure pepper, and herbs compliment a sandwich as well as sauces you are used to using. You can add them back in a few weeks if you wish. (See Appendix G - Recipes)*

• *Be careful to use only homemade dressings, avoiding commercial buttermilk as a base. (Buttermilk is made using enzymes to sour the milk and usually contains carrageenan). Olive oils, organic (unsulfered) vinegar or lemon with spices to your taste is a nice addition to your salad or vegetable sandwich. Wine vinegars may contain added sulfite. (See Appendix G - Recipes)*

Even "natural or organic" dressings containing ingredients such as xanthum gum, guar gum and carrageenan, which may effect you.

• *Try eating chunky vegetable salads instead of salads full of lettuce. Spice them up with salt, pepper and garlic with a touch of oil and lemon. You might also avoid iceberg lettuce, as it will inherently produce extra mucous in your digestive system and additional problems. Try romaine, green or red leaf, or alfalfa sprouts (high in proteins) as a salad base instead.*

If you carefully read labels and follow the suggestions we have put together you will eliminate most forms of free glutamic acid you may have been ingesting. Here's some other ways to avoid ingesting free glutamic acid.

- *Never combine fermented items with proteins. One can combine with the other to form free glutamic acid during cooking. (ie: vinegars, soy, marinades, etc with meat).*

- *Don't eat overcooked meat and poultry products. Over cooking leads to hydrolization and breaks down protein potentially freeing glutamic acid. Forget those crock pot meals and look for quick, 30 minute or less recipes using as little processing as possible.*

- *Other than hamburger or other ground meats and poultry, lean meats are best eaten rare or medium rare. The reason that many suggest eating only well-done ground meats is that during processing, surface bacteria can be mixed into the center of ground meats. Cooking it full through will help to kill these foreign bacteria.*

Unless your solid muscle meats (steaks, chops, etc) have been adulterated during handling or have parasites, rare or medium rare meats are fine to eat.

A special note about poultry and other proteins: you may have noticed a gelatin substance that appears hours after portions of cooked poultry, fish or meat has been let to stand and cool. This material is quite natural, as are the "pan juices" we all use to create gravies, marinades and sauces from, however, these natural juices may also contain free glutamic acid which can accumulate over time in leftovers. Eat animal and fowl proteins right after preparation. Only make enough for one meal for the first couple of weeks. Start experimenting with eating "left over" portions in your menu plans later.

• *Never use poultry, beef or pork broth as a base to steam vegetables or rice. Poultry, beef and pork stock is high in free glutamic acid, even if home made from organically range-fed and raised sources. (See Appendix G - Recipes, for a vegetable base stock)*

• *If you feel you are extremely sensitive to MSG, avoiding all poultry products may be in your favor. (solid and ground meats, broth and gravies made from pan drippings included) Remove it from your meal plans for the first few weeks and add the poultry products back in your diet to challenge yourself later. You will be able to tell how well you tolerate it after this exercise.*

• *A good substitute for animal protein is fish, frozen packaged fish or fresh from the butcher. There are a few brands of canned tuna on the market, usually available in "natural or organic" stores that are packaged using only water. Avoid those with salt, broth, hydrolyzed protein or other "ingredients".*

• *Never over cook vegetables. Light steaming helps to keep the nutrients intact. Vegetables also contain proteins that can hydrolyze and ferment causing glutamic acid to be freed. Over cooked or canned tomatoes, peas and mushrooms are particularly suspect.*

• *Avoid all packaged solid, string, shredded or grated cheeses during the first few weeks. Commercially available cheese may have been processed using enzymes, rennet (protein derived from the stomach lining of the animal) and dyes*

Organics

If you can't find organic milk and dairy products, try to remove dairy from your diet for the first few weeks, adding only whole milk and butter products back later. To insure that the dyes used to make cheese yellow or orange are not suspect items, use only white cheeses first, adding colored cheese later. (All cheese is really white by nature. Annatto and other food colorants are used to make it orange or yellow to suit you "visually".)

If you have no organic food suppliers in your area, you may consider having foods mail ordered to you. A good source is the World Wide Web addresses listed in the Appendices (see Appendix A).

If you don't have a computer at home to access the World Wide Web, there are generally ones available, for limited or no charge at your public library. They will usually provide a printer near by to let you print your information to take with you for later use.

Water ...

Of course water is an important part of any healthy diet, but during an elimination diet it is essential. Six to eight glasses (8oz) daily will help you to digest and eliminate not only the foods you are consuming, but also help you process and eliminate residual toxins and "garbage" out of your system. This is an important aspect of your success and helps to rehydrate your skin, digestive tract and cleanse your organs during your elimination.

Unfortunately, you also need to check the labels of your water sources. You might think twice about drinking or cooking with tap water as it can potentially contain chlorine, lead, and fluoride. Some bottled "drinking" waters may have added salts and minerals. Bottled spring or distilled water is best.

Eating out ...

When I first started trying to eat out (I travel more than 50% of the time), not being able to find things to eat off of the menu would reduce me to tears. Instead of letting it get the better of me, I decided to fight back. I am now very outspoken at restaurants of how my food needs to be prepared and carry a copy of the suspect items with me to give to wait staff and kitchen help.

I don't frequent restaurant chains where foods are generally prepared in bulk and sold to local owners or management. Many times meats and poultry are treated with marinades containing free glutamic acid or other preservative agents prior to reaching the local restaurant location. Food staff may not be aware of this preparation and unknowingly tell you that their meats are safe for your consumption. (Meats, poultry and fish are especially suspect unless provided from an organic source and handled with the utmost care in preparation and packaging for shipment).

I will most often find a small diner or cafe where I can speak with the staff directly and we can talk about how to make a meal I can truly enjoy. Organic and vegetarian restaurants usually have the largest selections and are great about special requests.

If the ingredient comes from a bottle, bag or box, I ask to see the ingredient list. I'm never shy about asking to speak with kitchen staff or management. The restaurant business is based upon service and quality; everyone I have ever approached was more than willing to help accommodate me.

Airline Food ...

Aside from the jokes "plane food" has endured for years about taste and appeal, there are numerous reasons to avoid it due to how it has had to be prepared. There's no practical value in going through the host of ingredients you might find in the food, again - just avoid it. Nuts, pretzels, snacks, all are heavily laden with items from our *Hidden Sources* lists. Pack your own snacks and meals and eat heartily!

Alcohol ...

Avoid alcohol during the first phases of the elimination. Not only does alcohol have a dehydrating (drying) effect upon the system, alcohol also contains many suspect trigger ingredients and impurities, as well as, having the aggravating affect of exacerbating the problems of the MSG sensitive person.

Yes, Exercise ...

Increase exercise! One of the largest organs you have is your skin. Its main purpose is to act as an elimination channel for excess toxins and byproducts your body needs to get rid of by sweating. One of the best ways to sweat is to exercise! If you aren't already taking brisk walks for 30 minutes at least 3 times a week, start now! Given you are capable, this will help increase your metabolism and aid in digestion and improved well being.

Going for the Gold ...

If you really want to get into a full elimination and detoxification program, here's a few great books to look into; *6 Weeks to a Toxic Free Body* by Dean D. Kimmel, *Diet for a New America* and *Diet for a New World* by John Robbins and *Diet for a Poisoned Planet* by David Steinman.

Each can help you to eliminate food additives and toxins in your diet and system, improving your health and well being, using more restrictive methods than following our modified elimination model. All of these books have great recipes, easily adapted to any regional taste. The appendices of the books are filled with directories on wholesale organic food resources, suppliers, natural hygiene practitioners, spas and consumer groups and organizations.

As with so many of the books on the market today, few speak to the new findings of the sufferers of MSG sensitivity. Incorporate the great teachings in these books with what you have learned here to your advantage.

The Feel Good Handbook

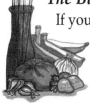

The Basics of a Full Elimination Diet...

If you were to be given an elimination diet by a medical practitioner, here are some of the basic elements and "rules" you might follow. You could use this as a model for foods to use for the next few weeks. You shouldn't see any negative results and may actual discover food allergies or sensitivities as you add back in poultry, beef, wheat and other products shortly. However, following along on any restrictive diet without the advice of an informed professional may lead you into a poorly balanced diet and you could suffer from malnutrition or other vitamin, mineral or substance deficiencies.

The difference between a full elimination diet and my suggested "modified elimination" is its "intensity and restrictiveness". A full elimination diet might last as long as 180 days or more. You will be asked to eliminate almost all food groups for the first few weeks and then add them back one at a time. (After eliminating eggs and dairy, you would have to prepare baked goods without benefit of milk, eggs, butters and fats until the time you could begin to add them back into your diet.)

Here are some of the basics of a full elimination program:
* *Focus menu planning around permissible items on the following food lists, rotate them so that you will not eat one item more than once in a four day period.*

* *Eliminate all dairy products and eggs*

* *Avoid meats, seafood and animal proteins and fats*

* *Eliminate gluten, wheat, barley, malt, oats, rye, corn and spelt products*

* *No caffeine, tobacco, processed sugar, sodas or alcohol*

* *Drink at least 2 quarts of pure water daily*

Full Elimination Diet Permissible Foods Chart

Asparagus	Potato flour
Broccoli	Potatoes
Brown Rice	Pumpkin
Carrots	Rice
Cane sugar	Rice flour
Celery	Safflower Oil
Sunflower Oil	Salmon (organic, range free)
Fresh garlic	Sea salt
Ginger	Sesame
Herb teas (no citrus or berry)	Soybeans (steamed)
Lamb (organic, range free)	Spinach
Lentils	Split peas
Lima beans	String Beans
Linseed oil	Sunflower seeds
Oatmeal	Sweet Potato
Olive Oil	Turnips
Parsley	Walnuts
Pears	Yams

Information with the permission of Yorkshire Labs.
http://www.yorkshire.co.uk/

After 2-3 weeks:

* *Add small portions of food back into your diet from the food groups; start with fruits, add vegetables, starches, carbohydrates, fish, meat, poultry, dairy, wheat, corn and nuts being last as they are generally suspect items in so many recipe items.*

* *Add only one item every 3-7 days.*

* *Watch and note any and all reactions, negative reactions may require you to eliminate those items permanently from your diet*

Daily for the next 2-3 weeks; consume reasonable amounts of the foods on the permissible list; vegetables, rice, potatoes, non-enriched pasta, gluten\wheat free breads, whole butter, vegetable based soups and plenty of water.

Information with the permission of Yorkshire Labs.
http://www.yorkshire.co.uk/

" *...adverse effects of MSG for me are:*
> *blurred vision*
> *muscle weakness & lack of coordination*
> *impaired immune system*
> *impaired thought processes*
> *skin rash*
> *migraine headaches (with very large doses)*

There are times when I get symptoms of MSG consumption and am unable to trace the source because of misleading labels on prepared foods. My symptoms also are dose related - worse when consuming pure MSG or larger amounts of hydrolyzed protein and other lesser sources. Discovering that MSG is "hidden" under other names on food labels, I was able to further eliminate MSG from my diet (hydrolyzed protein, sodium caseinate, autolyzed yeast, yeast extract, natural flavoring, malted barley, etc..."

Excerpts from a letter on file at the FDA

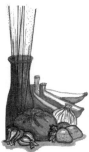

Time for a Reality Check ...

Two or three weeks after beginning your
modified elimination, take some time to
reflect on what has happened over the past few
weeks before you start to add items back
into your diet.

Have you made the best attempt possible to eat unadulterated
foods? Have you eliminated all forms of MSG? Are you getting
enough rest and exercise? Are you consuming plenty of water?

Make an honest assessment of where you are now. Are you
experiencing fewer bouts with gas, intestinal distress,
headaches, dizziness, mood swings, twitches, tingling, and
muscle aches or joint pain? Is your complexion clearer, have
you experienced a loss of weight; is an increase in your stamina
evident?

Included in many of the benefits is a sense of well being and
self worth that comes from your ability to control how you feel
after a meal. I personally have benefited by enjoying

> Improved digestion and assimilation of food
> Improved look and feel to my skin and complexion
> Improved weight control and weight management
> Improved balance of moods and anxiety

As you add food items back into your diet, do so consciously!

Eat the new item and note ANY change you experience within
minutes, hours or days. If the reaction is a negative one - you
may want to avoid these items altogether.

Meal and Reaction Form

Day _____ Date_____

Meal _____ Time _____ **AM PM**

Description: _____

_____

_____

_____

_____

Any reactions: _____Yes _____ No

Date/Time Noticed: _____

Description: _____

_____

_____

_____

Photo copy for your continued use. One per meal.
Three will fit on one 8.5 in x 11 in. page.

Phase Two: *Reintroducing Foods and Other Products ...*

Start off by introducing only one item at a time into your meal plan. This is extremely important if you are to truly sense any changes from specific products. My recommendation is to remain on the basic routine and add organic forms of these foods first, migrating to commercial brands you have used in the past (given they do not contain a source of MSG).

Note Your Reactions ...

See which fruit, vegetable, dairy, and then meat products you tolerate well. Every 3-5 days, you can begin to add one new item in that order. As you reintroduce foods, maintain a diary of not only the foods you eat but also the potential reactions that may occur. Your goal is to identify which types and sources of free glutamic acid you are prone to show sensitivity reactions from eating or using.

Reactions Can Vary ...

You may find, as I did, that different types of free glutamic acid produce a variety of reactions. Some of the reactions matched while others were completely dissimilar.

For me, modified food starch, cornstarch, hydrolyzed proteins (especially from corn products) make me extremely tired, listless and moody. My body has muscle and joint aches and I often feel disassociated and "hazy"; its hard to function coherently and I often feel "drunk" or "drugged" and unable to control even the most basic human functions such as sleep. After ingestion of the above I've been known to drop off into a sound sleep unable to be roused for hours. I often wake from these induced sleeps feeling like I have a "hangover" and find it hard to get up and going again.

Ingestion of monosodium glutamate specifically causes my heart to race; I feel anxious and ready to climb the walls if confined in a small room. My joints and muscles ache and often twitch uncontrollably; so too, do my eye lids; I get immediate dry mouth and find that my skin feels flushed and "tighter" or dry too; loud ringing in my ears, headaches and migraines are also common. The ingredient monosodium glutamate causes me to experience vomiting, nausea along with a royal dose of gastrointestinal distress in the form of gas; diarrhea; bouts of colitis (severe enough at times to have forced me into colonic therapy).

Processed soy products, tofu, and gums or thickeners like xanthum gum, guar gum and maltodextrin give me gas and bloating. Breads laden with malted barley and enriched flours, especially with L-cysteine added give me gas and induce a thick mucous laden stool or diarrhea. These maladies may last for a few hours, days or longer.

Like most people, I retain water and have been known to gain up to 7 pounds of water weight in the matter of hours after ingesting foods containing any form of MSG.

If I mix them all together in a meal, including carbonated sodas or juice containing citric acid or aspartame, I'm sick for a week.

Symptom relief ...

In the event you find that you have reactions du
you begin your modified elimination, there is anecdotal
evidence that daily supplements can help to minimalize your
distress from MSG.

Supplements of magnesium, Vitamin B6, and/or Vitamin C
(from natural sources that do not contain fillers, starch, yeast
or preservatives) have been suggested. These may not work
for everyone.

The most valuable skill you can acquire is being able to
"listen" to your body. Don't ignore minor aches and pains,
they are indicators that you may be "building up" MSG in
your system and "weighing" it down, hampering your ability
to feel good. Should you continue to ignore the symptoms,
you may find yourself in a situation where you may have a
"full blown" reaction.

I find that plenty of pure water and rest can help ease my
symptoms. I will also be extremely careful of what I eat for the
next few days if I have a reaction, to let my system "rest" and
recover. It is VERY important that you give your body time to
"heal" from a reaction.

"MSG has almost ruined my life. It definitely has impaired it. I haven't driven or worked for over 8 years. I have been completely dependent upon my family. I hate not being able to go out, get in my car and just go to the store. The Grand Mal Seizures [I experienced] are under control now that I avoid MSG. But excluding MSG from my diet completely has been impossible because of the deceptive food labels."

"My husband and I read every label of every product I eat, but so many companies try to hide MSG by hiding[it] under other names [that] it is very confusing. If I ingest MSG within several hours my heart races so fast it becomes ineffective and I have to take a heart pill..."

"If there isn't anything wrong with MSG, why do food manufacturers go to such trouble to cover up and use other names on the labels instead of MSG[?]."

"To say that MSG limits my enjoyment of life is putting it mildly."

Excerpts from letters on file at the FDA

Phase Three:
Living a MSG FREE Lifestyle

Read Labels

From here, you will no doubt be a great deal more conscious of what may be causing your symptoms. You have hopefully kept a detailed diary of food items and your reactions to refer to and can pin point suspect items easily.

Keep reading labels. Food distributors and manufactures can change the ingredients on labels at their own whim. Further investigation and understanding of label information will go a long way to helping you to remain MSG FREE.

Label Dictionaries and Additive Guides

Nutrient label claim definitions are starting to appear on the book shelves for consumers. Written for the lay person, these guides attempt to define and categorize food additives and ingredients for the consumer. A word of caution, as these books often do not address free glutamic acid(MSG), autolyzed yeast or hydrolyzed proteins and their MSG content. In fairness to them, much of this information has only recently been disclosed.

I found the following books to be of help in understanding what is in the foods I eat, though none adequately cover the subject of MSG. *The Pocket Guide to Good Food* by Margaret M. Wittenberg, adds seasonal buying guides, storage suggestions and expanded sampling of the types of processes and additives that our foods are subject to and may contain. *The Pocket Dictionary of Food Additives*, by J. Michael Lapchick and two other books that add dimension to this information are *Foods that Harm, Foods that Heal* by Reader's Digest and *The Nutritional Bible* by Jean Anderson, MS and Barbara Deskins,

Ph.D., RD. Again, using both The Feel Good Handbook and these guides, you can learn more about the additives in the foods you prepare for you and your family to eat.

Examples of Misleading labels ...

I frequent a grocery store that has locations around the country and claims not to carry any items on their shelves that contain monosodium glutamate, food additives or preservatives. I have shopped here for years, but found that I often picked up items that made me ill after eating them.

Now that I know it's the free glutamic acid that causes me problems, I look carefully at ALL labels. This store's corporate advertised "No MSG" policy had lulled me into believing that all the products on their shelves should be safe for me to use. As the following examples prove, that is not the case. Also, its important to remember that the California Organic Food Act does NOT identify standards for the use of hydrolyzed vegetable proteins or autolyzed yeast products. Nor does the USDA regulate for their use on meat items. YOU MUST ASK the producer specifically! It goes back to consumer knowledge. Keep your *Hidden Sources* lists handy as you shop; any where you shop!

(Suspect Sources of MSG <u>underlined</u> and **bold**)

YAYA Cheese Popcorn
Organic Air Popped Popcorn, Canola Oil, Cheddar cheese (milk, cheese culture, salt, **<u>enzymes)</u>** whey, sea salt, **<u>buttermilk</u>**

Organic Gourmet Vegetable Bouillon
Sea Salt, **<u>nutritional yeast extract</u>**, non-hydrogenated palm, oil, vegetables (carrots, leeks, celery, onions, bell peppers), **<u>spices</u>**, parsley

Tofu-Rella (cheese substitute)

Organic tofu (water, soybeans, calcium sulfate), **caseinate** (milk protein), soy oil, **modified food starch**, garlic, **spice**, sodium citrate, salt, **citric acid**, sorbic acid, vitamins and minerals (various)

Dr. McDougall's Smart Cups (various flavors)
Vegetarian Split Pea & Barley

Pre-cooked split green peas, barley, **natural flavor**, dehydrated vegetables (carrots, potatoes, celery), onion, **potato starch**, **autolyzed yeast extract**, garlic, **spices**, and unrefined sea salt.

East Coast West Low Fat Cream Cheese

Lite cream cheese (pasteurized cream, cheese culture, **carob bean gum**, **guar gum**, red & green peppers, carrot, radish, green onion, parsley

Pacific Rice Non-Dairy Rice Drink (milk substitute)

Filtered water, brown rice, tricalcium phosphate, lactobacillus acidolphilus and L. Bifidus cultured product added, **guar gum**, **xanthum gum**, **carregeenan**, Vitamin A Palmitate & Vitamin D_2.

Mayacamas - Hollandaise Sauce (and others)

Unbleached wheat flour, **whey powder**, **natural lemon flavor**, dried egg yolk, paprika, **natural vinegar flavor**, **spices**, **guar gum**.

Consumer Advocacy ...

A consumer advocacy group that is working diligently against fraudulent labeling practices is the Truth in Labeling Campaign (TLC). On December 13, 1994, a citizens' petition was filed with the US Department of Health and Human Services, FDA, to require that MSG (free glutamic acid) must be clearly labeled when used in foods.

The FDA chose to ignore this initial petition so suit against the FDA was filed. For the most updated information, refer to the Truth in Labeling Campaign web site or contact them at their mailing address (listed in the appendix).

Consumer Education and Support ...

The National Organization Mobilizing to Stop Glutamate (NO MSG) provides educational and support opportunities to interested parties. They have a robust newsletter focusing on industry news and developments, legislation, education, meal planning, recipes and networking. NO MSG has just completed their second conference and plan to continue these events annually. NO MSG also has a web site and contact information in the appendix.

Consumer Protection ...

A letter written on December 5, 1991 by Janice F. Oliver, Director of the Office of Regulatory Guidance, Center for Food Safety and Applied Nutrition, FDA, defines the responsibilities of a food provider in listing ingredients in their wares. It states;

> "a food label that declares 'No MSG Added' is false and misleading under section 403 (a)(1) of the Federal Food, Drug, and Cosmetic Act when the label also lists any hydrolyzed protein as an ingredient since it contains MSG."

False and misleading labels are illegal. It is appropriate to ask your grocer not to carry these products, and to report them to the office of the:

FDA Commissioner
(301-827-2410 or 301-827-5930 fax)

or to your local FDA office as well as to the Consumer Fraud Division of your State Attorney General.

If you also want to help with the cause of insuring that MSG is noted correctly on labels and that public funding is made available for its study, please write to your legislator about your thoughts and experiences. In California, for example, a note to our senator can be of a great deal of value as legislative action is normally done at the insistence of constituents. Californians, please write to:

The Honorable Dianne Feinstein
United States Senate
Washington, DC 20510

Fraudulent Labels ...

The following examples of false and misleading labels with examples of ingredients that contain MSG were collected in 1995. Trademarks and tradenames are those of their owners.

Producer	Product Name	Statement	Free Glutamate
A Taste of Thai	Spicy Thai Peanut Bake	"No MSG Added"	Hydrolyzed vegetable protein
Modern Products	The Original Spike All Purpose Seasoning	"No MSG Added"	Flavor yeast; Hydrolyzed protein
Live Food Products	Bragg Liquid Aminos	"No MSG"	Glutamic acid
Campbell's Soup	Franco American TeddyOs Pasta with Tomato & Cheese Sauce	"No MSG"	Enzyme modified butter; Enzyme modified cheddar cheese
Campbell Soup	Franco American SpaghettiOs: Pasta with meatballs in tomato sauce	"No MSG"	Enzyme modified cheddar cheese; Enriched bread crumbs; Enzyme modified butter; Citric acid; Nonfat dry milk

Producer	Product Name	Statement	Free Glutamate
Lipton	Kettle Creations Soup Mix Bean Medley with Pasta	"No MSG Added"	Yeast extract; Maltodextrin; Natural flavors
Trader Joe's	Northwest Territory Premium Beef Stew	"No MSG Added"	Autolyzed yeast extract; Natural flavorings
Campbell's	Healthy Request New England Clam Chowder	"No MSG"	Modified Food Starch;Guar Gum Whey Protein Concentrate, Maltodextrin
Campbell's	Healthy Request Chicken Broth	"No MSG"	Chicken stock; Chicken flavor; Flavoring
Campbell's	Healthy Request Cream of Chicken Soup	"No MSG"	Modified food starch; Maltodextrin
Chef Boyardee	Sesame Street Pasta Shapes in Tomato and Meat Sauce	"No MSG"	Maltodextrin; Flavorings; Enzyme modified cheese

What's left to eat?

There is A LOT! Just shop and cook wisely. We try to stick to a diet of fresh organic fruits, produce, starches, dairy, meats and fish. We all have a different set of tolerance levels so each of us have different needs. It's all about moderation and knowing your body. (I may avoid things my husband and son may not.)

The following is a list of few example items from our own cupboard.Those items noted with (*) may sell multiple varieties of products and one or more may contain added ingredients with MSG. We included some recipes are in Appendix G. **Trademarks and tradenames are those of their owners.**

Annie's Cupboard ....

Breads, Chips, Cookies, Rice, Pasta & Stuff
Carr's Crackers (they have a wide variety)
Eden Foods Vegetable Alphabets (noodles)
Whole Foods 365 Organic Pasta and Noodles (various)
Giusto's Vita-Grain Breads (wonderful array of choices!)
Whole Foods Tortillo Chips (no flavorings)
Ya Ya's Plain Popcorn(cheese flavors may contain enzymes)*
Old Fashioned Quaker Oats (5 min) (Instant & flavored)*
Brent and Sam's Cookies*
Lundberg Family Farms Rice(Risotto & pilaf mix have MSG)*
Waffle Heaven (mixed varieties of frozen waffles)

Canned Soups, Sauces & Tomato Products
Muir Glen Tomato Products & Sauces*
Health Valley Organic Soups *
Bearitos (whole & refried beans)*

Dairy
Organic Valley Butter (salted or not)
Organic Valley Eggs
Horizon Organic Whole Milk*
Breyers Ice Cream *

Frozen Veggies
C & W Frozen Vegetables

Other
Domino Cane Sugar
Tuna Fish (either Whole Foods 365 Brand or most organic
    brands in oil or water with NO additives)
Bacon - no added preservatives, nitrates or sulfates (we use
    Beeler's brand, although it is colored using beet powder,
    this may effect those extremely sensitive to MSG)*
Rice Dream* (milk substitute)

In conclusion...

I hope that after you complete the modified elimination and continue to monitor what you eat that you will begin experiencing the benefits of a reduction in the amount of free glutamic acid in your diet.

If you feel that you are not getting full benefit, explore the appendices for more information of other items that may be causing you reactions. The appendices also contain support groups and organizations, informative Web sites, books and medical reference materials that may be able to help you along the way.

You're welcome to mail me with comments or questions (and we are always looking for great recipes, tips and suggestions to share with others.

You can email me at Annie@thelighthousepress.com or write c/o The LightHouse Press, 3555 South El Camino Real, # 301, San Mateo, Ca 94403.

The LightHouse Press also has a web site that contains all sorts of up to date information and other links to web sites of interest. You can sign our guest book and request information from one of the many groups listed on the site too. The address for the site is www.msgfree.com or www.thelighthousepress.com

Be well.

oh, by the way...

Tag! You're IT!

Appendices

The Feel Good Handbook

Appendix A
Information on the World Wide Web (WEB)

Related Web Sites

Use Excite®, HOTBOT®, Lycos®, Yahoo® or other search engines to find more information on the WEB. Key words that may help are: "monosodium glutamate", "food additives", "organic", "alternative health", or use specific words related to your interest: (ie. asthma, ADD, heart condition, salt, Parkinson's, Alzheimer's, etc). Don't stop at the first few sites! You may find your best information a number of "pages" into the search results.

MSG Related:

http://
members.aol.com/adandjack/truthinlabeling.htm
http://www.annapolis.net/members/holland
http://www.tiac.net/users/mgold/msg/msg.html
http://www.msgfree.com
http://www.nomsg.com
http://home.earthlink.net/~recruiting/msg.html

Allergy Related:

http://www.yorkshire.co.uk/allergy
http://alt.medmarket.com
http://www.allergyconnection.com
http://www.ivanhoe.com
http://www.vegweb.com/wwwboard/health
http://world.std.com/~ephraim

Elimination Diet Related:

http://www2.skyisland.com/skyisland/recipes
http://www.rocketcity.com/doctors/elimination.htm
http://www.accessible.com.au/handbook/
elimdiet.htm

Other Misc. Related:

http://www.tiac.net/users/mgold
http://www.TheLightHousePress.com
http://www.lung.ca

Commerce on the WEB - Buying Online:

Online commerce is as easy as shopping from a catalog these days. You will have the same type of payment options (credit card, checks, mail in orders) and the ease of browsing as many store fronts as any giant mall. Secure transactions on the net, policy and procedures are normally well defined at each site.

Use a search engine like HOTBOT® or Lycos® to locate sites on the WEB: I used the word "organic", looked for "food resellers" and found these vendors and distributors online. Remember to ask them if they use "hydrolyzed proteins, sodium caseinate or autolyzed yeast" ingredients in their products - not just "monosodium glutamate" or "MSG".

Bandana's	Cedar Hill Seasonings
The Diet Shoppe	Landreth Farms Wild Rice
Mediterranean Delights	Prunotto Farms

Free Info Online:
www.TheLightHousePress.com **or** www.MSGFree.com

You can browse our publisher's site by using either of the above URLs. Here you will find links to the previously mentioned sites, as well as others added since printing; you will also find *Books for Sale* that are listed (if in print) within the following appendix section. The site also has information on both Truth in Labeling Campaign and NO MSG.

"Glutamate Industry" Sites
Two industry sites will appear in most of the responses to your search requests. Both *The Glutamate Association* and The *International Food Information Council* (IFIC). It's important to review these sites to see how these groups promote the use and legitimization of MSG, monosodium glutamate and other excitotoxins. Remember *"Rule One"*. Read with caution.

Appendix B
Recommended Reading

Books are available for sale on The LightHouse Press web site for up to 40% off through AMAZON.COM.

In Bad Taste:
The MSG Syndrome
George R. Schwartz, M. D.
Santa Fe: Health Press, 1988
(ISBN #0-29173-00-7)

Excitotoxins:
The Taste That Kills
Russell L. Blaylock, M. D.
Santa Fe: Health Press, 1994
(ISBN #0-929173-14-7)

Aspartame (NutraSweet):
Is it Safe?
H. J. Roberts, M. D.
Philadelphia: Charles Press,
1990
(ISBN #0-914993-580)

6 Weeks to a Toxic-Free Body
Dean D. Kimmel:
Corbin House Pub
(ISBN 0-9621446-2-2)

Bittersweet Aspartame -
A Diet Delusion
Barbara Mullarkey;
NutriVoice c1992
708-848-0116

Diet for a New America; and
Diet for a New World
John Robbins;
(ISBN:0-380-71901-0)

Diet for a Poisoned Planet
David Steinman;
(ISBN:0-345-37465-7)

Pocket Dictionary of
Food Additives
J. Michael Lapchick:
(ISBN:1-56561-027-x)

Fit For Life
Harvey & Marilyn Diamond;
Warner Books; c1985
(ISBN: 0-446-51322-9)

Heavenly Feasts
Arcia M. Kelly;
Bell Tower, NYC
(ISBN: 0517-88522-0

Pocket Guide to Good Food
Margaret M. Wittenberg
(ISBN: 0-89594-747-1)

*The New Book of
Food Combining*
Jan Dries; Element: c1992
(ISBN: 1-85230-599-9)

*Why Can't My Child
Behave?*
Feingold Assoc.
JH001
ph # 516-369-9340

Sweet'ner Dearest
H. J. Roberts, MD
The Sunshine Sentinel Press,
West Palm Beach, FL, c1992

*Foods That Harm
Foods that Heal*
Readers Digest; c1996
(ISBN 0-895577-912-9)

*Why Your Child is
Hyperactive*
Feingold Assoc.
RH734262
call: 516-369-9340

*The Bitter Truth About
Artificial Sweeteners*
by Dennis Remington, MD
and Barbara Higa, RD
Vitality House International,
Provo, UT, c1987

*Encyclopedia of Nutrition
& Good Health*
Robert A. Ronzio;Facts on
File, Inc.;
(ISBN 0-8160-2665-3)

Appendix C
Organizations & Support Groups

Aspartame Consumer Safety Network (1987)
P. O. Box 990634
Dallas, Texas 75399
Marystod@airmail.net
URL:http://web2.airmail.net
(800) 969-6050
(214) 352-4268

Celiac Disease Foundation
13251 Ventura Blvd, Ste 300
Studio City, CA 91604
818-990-2354

EPA Safe Water Hotline
401 M Street SW
Washington, DC 20460
800-426-4791

Feingold Association (FAUS)
P.O. Box 6550
Alexandria, VA 22306
703-768-FAUS

Mission Possible
P. O. Box 28098
Atlanta, Georgia 30358
betty@pd.org

Mothers and Others for Pesticide Limits
P.O. Box 96048
Washington, DC 20077

NO MSG
P.O. Box 367
Santa Fe, New Mexico 87504
800-BEAT-MSG

Nutrition for Optimal Health Association (NOHA)
P.O. Box 380
Winnetka, IL 60093

The Pure Food Campaign
1130 17th Street, NW, Ste 300
Washington DC 20036
800-253-0681
202-775-1132

Truth in Labeling Campaign (TLC)
P. O. Box 2532
Darien, IL 60561
312-642-9333
adandjack@aol.com

Appendix D

Sensitivity to Salicylate and Benzoic Acid ...

There are other natural or synthetic substances that may cause sensitivity reactions. Salicylate sensitivity (aspirin allergy) is common and is believed to contribute to many health related and behavioral problems that are parallel to those that are found with MSG Sensitive people.

(Information from Feingold Association Literature - see Appendix C.)

Salicylate Sensitivity Common Reactions:

Skin
Increased tear secretion
Reddening of the eyes and
face

Ears
Ringing in the ears
(tinnitus)

Neurological
Depression
Mood swings

Skeletal
Joint paint of arthtalgia
Joint swelling
Muscular
Eye muscle disorders

Other Physical Symptoms
Bladder incontinence
Bleeding and inflamed
digestive tract

(Continued)
Chronic fatigue
Constipation or diarrhea
Forehead pressure
Mental and physical
sluggishness
Sensations of swelling
Sleep apnea - stops
breathing during sleep
Thirst, stinging, hot flashes
Upset stomach -

Cognitive and Perceptual Disorders
Inability to concentrate
Short attention span
Behavioral deficits
Distractibility
Fidgetiness
Nervousness
Poor self image
Temper flare-ups
Workaholism

91

Naturally Occurring Salicylate Acid

The following is a list of foods and products that contain specified "levels" of salicylate acid. To determine if you are salicylate or benzoic acid sensitive, remove these items initially from your diet and then reintroduce them as a challenge. For support and more current information, please contact Feingold Association (see Appendix C).

Almonds	high	Kumquat	low
Apples	high	Lemons	low
Apricots	high	Limes	low
All berries	high	Loquats	low
Aspirin	high	Papaya	low
Avocado	med	Persimmon	low
Banana	med	Watermelon	low
Bread fruit	low	Mango	low
Cantaloupe	low	Passion fruit	low
Casaba melon	low	Pears	low
Crenshaw melon	low	Pomegranate	low
Cherries	high	Rhubarb	low
Cloves	high	Nectarines	high
Cider	high	Oil of wintergreen	high
Cider vinegar	high	Oranges	high
Coffee	high	Peaches	high
Cucumbers	high	Peppers	high
Currants	high	Plums	high
Dates	high	Prunes	high
Fig	low	Tangerines	high
Honeydew melon	low	Tea	high
Grapes	high	Tomatoes	high
Grapefruit	med	Wine	high
Guava	high	Wine vinegar	high
Kiwi	low		

Naturally occurring Benzoates (benzoic acid)

Benzoic acids, like salicylates, can be found in some foods naturally. These are foods that contain naturally occurring benzoic acid and can aggravate or mock the reactions of MSG and salicylate sensitivity. Again, to determine sensitivity to them, incorporate their elimination and challenge into your plan

Bananas	Greengage plums
Blueberries	Green peas
Broccoli	Licorice extract
Cauliflower	Pineapple
Cinnamon	Ripe olives
Cranberries	Spinach
Ginger	Tea
Green grapes	White potatoes

The Feel Good Handbook

Appendix E
Other Food Additives to Avoid ...

Aspartame (NutraSweet®), Cyclamates

Aspartame, an excitotoxin like MSG, causes brain lesions and neuroendocrine disorders in laboratory animals virtually identical to those caused by MSG. It is also known to cause human adverse reactions, some that are identical to those caused by MSG. The patents which have protected the original manufacturer (NutraSweet®) from competition are no longer valid. A host of "aspartame", NutraSweet®, knock off products will no doubt soon be available on the market under a variety of names. Refer to Appendix B for recommended reading.

Bovine Somatotropin

A genetically engineered recovinant Bovine Growth Hormone (rBGH) also known as Bovine Somatotropin or BST has recently found its way into the commercial production of dairy items. rBGH or BST is used as a supplement in a cow's diet and stimulates their milk production. Cow's injected with rBGH may suffer from increased udder infections (matitis), severe reproductive problems, digestive disorders, food and leg ailments and persistent sores and lacerations about their teats and milk system.

The administration of rBGH or BST weakens the cows overall stamina to fight off infection and illness, increasing the need for antibiotics and other drugs to fight increased disease. This may lead to greater risk of antibiotic and chemical contamination of milk and an increase in the resistance to antibiotics by the milk-drinking public.

Organic standards do not allow the use of rBGH or BST if the product is labeled "Organic". In other products, identifying rBGH or BST laden products can only be done by requesting "written assurance" that products are free of these substances. A group known as "The Pure Food Campaign", listed in the appendix, can supply you more current information. (See Appendix C.)

Typical Food Additives and Their Use

There are two groups of food additives to watch out for in our food, incidental additives and intentional additives. Along with MSG, artificial salicylic acid, and added benzoic acid, here's a list of some of the intentional additives often found in foods we eat everyday that can cause adverse reactions to those that are sensitive to them.

These items are mostly used to extend the shelf life of processed foods. Artificial colors, sweetners, flavoring agents are used to either mask lower quality, highly processed foods or "enhance" the flavor remaining in processed foods.

Artificial Sweeteners: (add sweetness to foods)
> Alitame
> Aspartame, aspartic acid
> Corn Syrup
> Corn Sweeteners

Artificial Flavorings\Flavoring Agents:
(Adds unique flavors to restore or enhance food flavor lost in processing)
> Petroleum Based
> Adipic Acid
> Ammoniated Glycyrrhizin
> Ammonium Sulfide
> Vanillin

Synthetic Artificial Colors: (made from petroleum)
> Synthetic Water Soluble-Certified by FDA: FD&C;
> Certified Synthetic Water-Insoluble colors:
> FD&C (Aluminum Lakes); suspected of being toxic
>> and carcinogenic

Pesticides(carcinogenic) :
Fungicides, herbicides, insecticides

Aldcarb	Opheny-phenol	Alachlor
Captafol	Permethrin	Metrolachlor
Captan	Chlordimeform	Oxadiazon
Maneb	Acephate	Oryzalin
Manczeb	Parathion	Pronamide
Folpet	Cypermethrin	Ethylfluralin
Chlorothalonil (Bravo)	Cyromazine	DiclofopMethyl
Metiram	Azinphos-ethyl	Terbutryn
Benomyl	Linuron	Glyphosate (RoundUp)

Preservatives, Anti Oxidant, Anti Mycotic and Acidulant Agents (keeps foods from spoiling, molds from growing or foods from oxidizing and changing colors):

Alpha-tocopherol (Vitamin E)
Alum (cake and patent)
Aluminum sulfate
Butylated hydroxyanisole
  (BHA)
Butylated hudoxytoluene
  (BHT)
Calcium disodium EDTA
Calcium propionate
Citric acid
Chlorine dips
Corn syrup
Disodium EDTA
Hydrogenated fats
Partially hydrogenated fats
Potassium benzoate
Potassium bisulfite
Potassium sorbate

Sodium benzoate
Sodium bisulfite
Sodium potassium
  metabisulfite
Sodium propionate
Sorbic acid
Sulfur dioxide
Sulfiting agents: sodium
  sulphite, sodium
  bisulphite,sodium
  metabisulphite and
  potassium metabisulphite)
Tertiary Butylhydroquinone
  (TBHQ)
Wax coatings (generally
found on fruits and
vegetables)

Dough conditioners, emulsifiers , enrichment, flavor enhancers and agents, fortifying, binders, acidulants, leavening agents, lubricants, maturing and bleaching agents, pH control agents, sequestrants, stablizers, texturizer, thickener, whipping agents: (products used to either improve consistancy, texture or stability of processed foods; enhance the flavor, nutritional value or appearance):

Azodiacarbonamide (ADA)
Agar
Alginates: ammonium
   alginate, calcium alginate,
   potassium alginate
Ammonium chloride
Ammonium bicarbonate
Ammonium phosphate
Ammonium sulfate
Bleached flours, rices
   (artificially aged)
Bromated flour
Brominated vegetable oil
Calcium disodium EDTA
Calcium peroxide
Carboxymethyl
   cellulose gum

Disodium EDTA
Disodium guanylate
Disodium inosinate
Irradiation
Hydrogenated fats
L-cysteine
Partially hydrogenated fats
Potassium bromate
Phosphates
Sodium nitrite
Sodium stearyol lactylate
Stearoyl-2-lactylate
Sodium diacetate
Vanillin

Fat Substitutes: (products used to simulate fats and butters used in recipes.)

> Appetize
> Caprein
> Guar Gum
> Hydrolyzed: protein, soy, oat, wheat, gluten
> Maltodextrin
> Olestra
> Starches: Modified Food Starch; Potato, Whey,
>   Soy, etc.
> Xanthum Gum

A special note about CORN Sensitivities:

For those that are definitely allergic to corn and corn products, the following may be of interest. As you may already be aware, corn syrup, cornstarch, etc, should all be avoided; on another note, the protein contained in corn, during processing, can cause the creation of free glutamic acid (MSG). Corn finds its way into all sorts of ingredients. Take note of this information on corn that was extracted from Ephraim's Home Pages at http://world.std.com/~ephraim

Another note: Most cola and soft drinks contain high amounts of corn syrup. Ephraim noted on his pages that foods marked "Kosher for Passover" are NOT supposed to contain any corn products for religious reasons and should be available during the holiday season.

- **Alcohol:** *check with manufacturers: vodka, beers and other alcoholic beverages may be made from corn products*
- **Baking powder**: *may contain cornstarch*
- **Bleached flour:** *may contain cornstarch*
- **Caramel Flavoring or Coloring**: *usually derived from corn syrup*
- **Citric Acid:** *is NOT always derived from citrus fruits, it is often derived from corn products*
- **Confectioner's Sugar**: *may contain cornstarch*
- **Dextrin:** *often derived from cornstarch*
- **Dextrose:** *often derived from corn (extremely common in intravenous solutions)*
- **Excipients:** *used as a binder or filler in tablets: may contain cornstarch*

- *Golden syrup:* generally found in baked goods; contains corn syrup
- *Invert Sugar or Syrup:* ensymatically treated corn sugars
- *Iodized Table Salt::* may contain dextrose
- *Malt, malt syrup, malt extract:* may be derived from corn, barley
- *Maltodextrin:* is derived from cornstarch
- *Mono and Di-glycerides:* made from animal and vegetable fats and oils; may be derived from corn
- *Sucrose:* may be derived from corn
- *Vanilla extract:* even real vailla extract may have corn syrup added
- *Xanthan gum:* fermantation of bacteriums and can often be cultured using corn sugars as a base

Appendix F
SELECTED REFERENCES ...

for the medical practitioner from *Monosodium Glutamate (MSG): References sufficient to demonstrate that MSG puts consumers at risk.*; Adrienne Samuels, Ph.D. - August 15, 1995

Allen, D. H. , Delohery, J. , & Baker, G. J. Monosodium L-glutamate-induced asthma. Journal of Allergy and Clinical Immunology. 80:No 4, 530-537, 1987.

Allen, D. H., and Baker, G. J. Chinese-restaurant asthma. N Engl JMed. 305: 1154-1155, 1981.

Anderson, S. A. , and Raiten, D. J. Safety of amino acids used as dietary supplements. Prepared for the Food and Drug Administration under contract No FDA 223-88-2124 by the Life Sciences Research Office, FASEB. July, 1992. Available from: Special Publications, FASEB, Rockville, MD.

Asnes, R. S. Chinese restaurant syndrome in an infant. Clin Pediat. 19: 705-706, 1980. Beal, M. F. Mechanisms of excitotoxicity in neurologic diseases. FASEB J. 6: 3338-3344; 1992.

Blaylock, R. L. Excitotoxins: The Taste that Kills Santa Fe,Health Press, 1994. Broadwell, R. D. , and Sofroniew, M. V. Serum proteins bypass the blood-brain fluid barriers for extracellular entry to the central nervous system. Exp Neurol. 120: 245-263, 1993.

Choi, D. W., and Rothman. S. M. The role of glutamate neurotoxicityin hypoxic-ischemic neuronal death. Annu Rev Neurosci. 13: 171-182, 1990.

Choi, D. W. Amyotrophic lateral sclerosis and glutamate-too much of a good thing? Letter. N Engl J Med. 326: 1493-1495, 1992.

Cochran, J. W. , and Cochran A. H. Monosodium glutamania: the Chinese Restaurant Syndrome revisited. JAMA. 252: 899, 1984.

Colman, A. D. Possible psychiatric reactions to monosodium glutamate. N Engl J Med. 299: 902, 1999.

During, M. J. , and Spencer, D. D. Extracellular hippocampal glutamate and spontaneous seizure in the conscious human brain. Lancet 341: 1607-1610, 1993.

Elman, R. The intravenous use of protein and protein hydrolysates. Ann New York Acad Sc. 47: 345-357, 1946.

Fisher, K. N. , Turner, R. A. , Pineault, G. , Kleim, J. , and Saari,M. J. The post weaning housing environment determines expression of learning deficit associated with neonatal monosodium glutamate(M. S. G.). Neurotoxicology and Teratology. 13(5):507-13, 1991.

Freed, D. L. J. and Carter, R. Neuropathy due to monosodium glutamate intolerance. Annals of Allergy. 48: 96-97, 1982. Frieder, B. and Grimm, V. E. Prenatal monosodium glutamate (MSG)treatment given through the mother's diet causes behavioral deficits in rat offspring. Intern J Neurosci. 23: 117-126, 1984.

Frieder, B. and Grimm, V. E. Prenatal monosodium glutamate. Neurochem. 48: 1359-1365, 1987. Gann, D. Ventricular tachycardia in a patient with the; Chinese restaurant syndrome; Southern Medical J. 70: 879-880,1977.

Gao, J. , Wu, J. , Zhao, X. N. , Zhang, W. N. , Zhang, Y. Y. , and Zhang,Z. X. [Transplacental neurotoxic effects of monosodium glutamateon structures and functions of specific brain areas of filialmice.] Sheng Li Hsueh Pao Acta Physiologica Sinica. 46(1):44-51,1994.

Gordon, W. P. Neurotoxic theory of infantile autism. In: Neurobiology of infantile autism. Proceedings of the International Symposium on Neurobiology of Infantile Autism, Tokyo, 10-11 November 1990.

Eds H. Naruse and E. M. Ornitz. Amsterdam: Excerpta Medica, 1992. Gore, M. E. , and Salmon, P. R. Chinese restaurant syndrome: fact orfiction. Lancet. 1(8162):251, 1980.

Kenney, R. A. The Chinese restaurant syndrome: an anecdote revisited. Fd ChemToxic. 24: 351-354, 1986.

Kenney, R. A. and Tidball, C. S. Human susceptibility to oral monosodium L-glutamate. Am J Clin Nutr. 25: 140-146, 1972.

Kubo, T, Kohira, R. , Okano, T. , and Ishikawa, K. Neonatal glutamate can destroy the hippocampal CA1 structure and impair discrimination learning in rats. Brain Research. 616: 311-314,1993.

Levey, S. , Harroun, J. E. and Smyth, C. J. Serum Glutamic acid levels and the occurrence of nausea and vomiting after intravenous administration of amino acid mixtures. J Lab ClinMed. 34: 1238-1248, 1949.

Lipton, S. A. , and Rosenberg, P. A. Excitatory amino acids as a final common pathway for neurologic disorders. N Engl J Med. 330: 613-622, 1994.

Lynch, J. F. Jr. , Lewis, L. M. , Hove, E. L. , and Adkins, J. S. Division of Nutrition, FDA, Washington, D. C. 20204. Effect ofmonosodium L-glutamate on development and reproduction in rats. Fed Proc. 29: 567Abs, 1970.

Lynch, J. F. , Jr. , Lewis, L. M. , and Adkins, J. S. (Division of Nutrition, FDA, Washington, D. C. 20204). Monosodium glutamate-induced hyperglycemia in weanling rats. J S Fed Proc. 31: 1477,1971.

Martinez F. , Castillo, J. Rodriguez, J. R. , Leira, R. , and Noya,M. Neuroexcitatory amino acid levels in plasma and cerebro spinal fluid during migraine attacks. Cephalalgia 13(2):89-93, 1993.

Neumann, H. H. Soup? It may be hazardous to your health. Am HeartJ. 92: 266, 1976.

Oliver. A. J. , Rich, A. M. , Reade, P. C. , Varigos, G. A. , and Radden,B. G. Monosodium glutamate-related orofacial granulomatosis. Review and case report. Oral Surg Oral Med Oral Pathol. 71: 560-564, 1991.

Olney, J. W. Excitotoxin mediated neuron death in youth and oldage. In: Progress in Brain Research, Vol 86, ed P. Coleman, G. Higgins, and C. Phelps, pp 37-51. New York: Elsevier, 1990.

Olney, J. W. Excitotoxic amino acids and neuropsychiatric disorders. Annu Rev Pharmacol Toxicol. 30: 47-71, 1990.

Olney, J. W. Excitatory amino acids and neuropsychiatric disorders. Biol Psychiatry. 26: 505-525, 1989.

Olney, J. W. , Ho, O. L. , and Rhee, V. Brain-damaging potential of protein hydrolysates. N Engl J Med. 289: 391-393, 1973.

Olney, J. W., Labruyere, J., and DeGubareff, T. Brain damage in mice from voluntary ingestion of glutamate and aspartate. Neurobehav Toxicol. 2: 125-129, 1980.

Olney, J. W. , Ho, O. L. Brain damage in infant mice following oral intake of glutamate, aspartate or cysteine. Nature. (Lond) 227:609-611, 1970.

Olney, J. W. Glutamate-induced retinal degeneration in neonatal mice. Electron-microscopy of the acutely evolving lesion. J Neuropathol Exp Neurol. 28: 455-474, 1969.

Olney, J. W. Brain lesions, obesity, and other disturbances in mice treated with monosodium glutamate. Science. 164: 719-721,1969.

Pohl, R. , Balon, R. , and Berchou, R. Reaction to chicken nuggets in a patient taking an MAOI. Am J Psychiatry. 145: 651, 1988.

Pradhan, S. N. , Lynch, J. F. , Jr. Behavioral changes in adult rats treated with monosodium glutamate in the neonatal state. Arch Int Pharmacodyn Ther. 197: 301-304, 1972.

Price, M. T. , Olney, J. W. , Lowry, O. H. and Buchsbaum, S. Uptake of exogenous glutamate and aspartate by circumventricular organs but not other regions of brain. J Neurochem. 36:1774-1990, 1981.

Ratner, D. , Esmel, E. , and Shoshani, E. Adverse effects of monosodium glutamate: a diagnostic problem. Israel J Med Sci. 20:252-253, 1984.

Reif-Lehrer, L. A questionnaire study of the prevalence of Chinese Restaurant Syndrome. Fed Proc. 36:1617-1623, 1977.

Reif-Lehrer, L. Possible significance of adverse reactions to glutamate in humans. Federation Proceedings. 35: 2205-2211, 1976.

Reif-Lehrer, L. and Stemmermann, M. B. Correspondence: Monosodium glutamate intolerance in children. N Engl J Med. 293: 1204-1205,1975.

Rothstein, J. D. , Martin, L. J. , and Kuncl, R. W. Decreased glutamate transport by the brain and spinal cord in amyotrophiclateral sclerosis. N Engl J Med. 326: 1464-1468, 1992.

Said, S. I. , Berisha, H. , and Pakbaz, H. NMDA receptors in the lung: activation triggers acute injury that is prevented by NO synthase inhibitor and by VIP. Society for Neuroscience Abstracts20:1994.

Samuels, A., Ph.D. Excitatory amino acids in neurologic disorders: letter to the editor. N Engl J Med. 331: 274-275, 1994.

Samuels, A. Ph.D. Monosodium L-glutamate: a double-blind study and review. Letter to the editor. Food and Chemical Toxicology. 31: 1019-1035, 1993.

Sathave, N. and Bodnar, R. J. Dissociation of opioid and nonopioid analgesic responses following adult monosodium glutamate pretreatment. Physiology and Behavior. 46: 217-222, 1989.

Sauber, W. J. What is Chinese restaurant syndrome? Lancet. 1(8170): 721-722, 1980.

Schainker, B. , and Olney, J. W. Glutamate-type hypothalamic-pituitary syndrome in mice treated with aspartate or cysteate in infancy. J Neural Transmission. 35: 207-215, 1974.

Schaumburg, H. H. , Byck, R. , Gerstl, R. , and Mashman, J. H. Monosodium L-glutamate: its pharmacology and role in the Chinese Restaurant Syndrome. Science. 163: 826-828, 1969.

Scher, W. , and Scher, B. M. A possible role for nitric oxide in glutamate (MSG)-induced Chinese restaurant syndrome, glutamate-induced asthma, 'Hot-dog headache', pugilistic Alzheimer's disease, and other disorders. Medical hypotheses. 38: 185-188,1992.

Schinko, I. In: Cerebrospinal flussigkeit-csf, ed D. Dommasch and H. G. Mertens, pp 66-99. Stuttgart: Thieme, 1980.

Schwartz, G. R. In Bad Taste: The MSG Syndrome. Santa Fe: HealthPress, 1988.

Scopp, A. L. MSG and hydrolyzed vegetable protein induced headache: review and case studies. Headache. 31:107-110, 1991.

Spencer, P. S. Guam ALS/Parkinsonism-dementia: a long-laten cyneurotoxic disorder caused by slow toxin(s) in food? Can JNeurol Sci. 14: 347-357, 1987.

Spencer, P. S. Environmental excitotoxins and human neurodegeneration. Conference on excitotoxic amino acids, London,November, 1991. (Peter S. Spencer, Center for research on occupational and environmental toxicology, Oregon Health Sciences University, Portland, Oregon 97201 USA)

Spencer, P. S. Western pacific ALS-Parkinsonism-dementia: A model of neuronal aging triggered by environmental toxins. In Parkinsonism and Aging, ed D. B. Calne, et al., pp 133-144. NewYork: Raven Press, 1989.

Spencer, P. S. , Ross, S. M. , Kisby, G. , and Roy, D. N. Western Pacific ALS: putative role of cycad toxins. In: AmyotrophicLateral Sclerosis: Current Clinical and Pathophysiological Evidence for Differences in Etiology, ed J. A. Hudson. Toronto: University of Toronto Press, 1990.

Spencer, P. S. Linking cycad to the etiology of western pacifica myotrophic lateral sclerosis. In: ALS. New Advances in Toxicology and Epidemiology, ed F. C. Rose and F. H. Norris. Smith-Gordon, 1990.

Spencer, P. S. Amyotrophic lateral sclerosis and other motor neuron diseases. In: Advances in Neurology, Vol 56, ed L. P. Rowland. New York: Raven Press, 1991. Squire, E. N. Jr. Angio-oedema and monosodium glutamate. Lancet. 988, 1987.

Appendix G
Selected Recipes ...

Most cooking starts with the basics, so here's a collection of a few of the recipes we use in our home.

Any recipe will do. Just steer clear of those that require the use of milk, soy, corn, fermented and yeast products during the beginning of your elimination. Be especially careful of using canned goods or prepared sauces (like Worstershire Sauce). Add these and other suspect ingredients back into your diet as you go. You can usually substitute unenriched flour for cornstarch in recipes and gravies to thicken them.

MSG Sensitivity is about dosage. I react to a small amount and tend to stay away from certain ingredients (such as chicken, corn and soy) that I don't tolerate well. Conversely, my husband seems to tolerate chicken and enjoys it freshly prepared several times a month. This just goes to show how everyone is different.

The recipes we included are just a place to begin. Most came from family members or friends and have been altered slightly, if possible, when they suggested an offending ingredient. I have yet to find a baking powder on the market without cornstarch as an ingredient so beware of using these ingredients or recipes that call for it until you rule out baking powder as a trigger for yourself. Incorporate what you have learned in the previous text and also review the section titled *Annie's Cupboard* for brand names of butter, milk, eggs, sugar and other ingredients that we use or experiment with your own regional brands.

Good Eating!

Order a copy of The Feel Good Handbook for friend or family member!

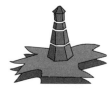

The LightHouse Press

You can: *5/00*
Call 888-298-1500 and order over the phone ...

•or•

Visit our website at
www.thelighthousepress.com or *www.msgfree.com*

•or•

You can photo copy or tear out & mail in this completed order form to:

The LightHouse Press
3555 W. El Camino Real, #301
San Mateo, CA 94403

Bill To: _____

Address: _____

City, State & Zip: _____

Day Time Phone: _____

Ship To: _____

Address: _____

City, State Zip: _____

The Feel Good Handbook
(ISBN 0-9662169-9-7)   ____ X $14.95 each _____
California Residents, please add 7.5% Sales Tax: _____
Shipping & Handling (US Post) $ 3.00
                    Total Due: _____

Credit Card # _____

Exp Date: _____

Account Name: _____

Billing Zip Code: _____

Signature: _____

Vegetable Stock ...

All commercial bouillon products I have found on store shelves has some type of MSG as an ingredient. If you enjoy soup, prepare a large batch of this stock and freeze it. That way it is always handy. (We use ice cube trays and then put the frozen stock cubes in freezer containers.)

- *Scrub all vegetables prior to preparation. You may peel carrots, etc if desired. Organic varieties preferred.*

- *Use 5-8 quart pan for preparation (non-aluminum)*

- *Use 3 quarts of water (preferably NOT tap water)*

- *Makes approximately 2 quarts of stock (unless reduced further) which will make approximately 72 cubes.*

Ingredients: *Butter - 2 tsp*
Carrots - 3 or 4 large (chopped)
Celery - 2 stalks (chopped)
Onion - 2 large (peeled and chopped)
Parsley - fresh 5 or 6 sprigs (dry - 2 to 3 tsp)
Bay leaf - 1/2 to 1 leaf
Thyme - fresh 1/2 tsp (1 tsp dry flakes)
Rosemary (optional) - fresh 1/2 tsp (1 tsp dry)
Garlic - to taste
 (2-3 large pieces diced or 1 tsp granuals)
Salt - 2 tsp (preferably pure sea salt)

- *Put the pot on over medium heat and melt butter. Add onions, celery, carrots and any other vegetables, saute until golden. This takes from 10 to 15 minutes.*

- *Add water and spices, cover and bring to boil. Reduce heat and simmer for 1 to 1.5 hour(s) or until the vegetables have "given up" their flavor to the broth. Strain. Store or serve.*

My Favorite Fish Soup...

- *Scrub all vegetables prior to preparation.
  (Organic varieties preferred.)*
- *Use appropriately sized sauce pan (non-aluminum)*
- *You can easily add other seafood to this dish if you tolerate them (Other varieties of fish, squid, mussels, shrimp, etc), be careful to select seafood not treated with sulfating agents*
- *Serves 4 as main dish (serve with rice & steamed veggies)*

Ingredients: *1 Quart Vegetable Stock (approx 32-36 ice cubes)
Lemon Grass - 1 tall stalk (cut to 1 inch pieces)
Celantro - 3 to 4 fresh sprigs (roughly chopped)
Jalapéno - 1 tsp (diced) [for HOT soup-1 medium]
Ginger - 1 to 1.5 inch fresh (sliced) or 1 tsp (dry)
Mushrooms - 3 to 4 large (sliced thinly)
1/2 to 1 pound firm fish, 2 inch cubes, slices
   (Cod, Halibut, Salmon, Tuna, etc.)
Salt and pepper - to taste*

- *Heat broth to below boiling and add fish, lemon grass, ginger. Steep for 5 to 10 minutes until fish is firm.*
- *Add remaining ingredients. Steep for 2 to 3 minutes and serve. You can also add pre-cooked rice before serving (1 to 2 cups).*

Steamed Pinion Nuts & Green Beans ...

Ingredients: *Use double boiler or steamer tray and sauce pan
Vegetable Stock - 1/4 cup or 2-3 Cubes or water
Pinion Nuts - 1/2 cup (whole)
Green Beans - 2 cups (cleaned)*

Heat vegetable stock or water, add beans and nuts, steam the green beans and pinion nuts for approximately 10 to 15 minutes. Pinion nuts should be warm through-out and beans darker green, but not over cooked. Serve hot, with butter and salt, if desired.

Mash Potato Soup...

- *You can easily add other vegetables to your taste with this recipe. It is a "mock cream of potato" soup.*

- *Scrub all vegetables prior to preparation. (Organic varieties preferred.)*

- *Use appropriately sized sauce pans (non-aluminum)*

- *Serves 4 as main dish (serve with salad and bread)*

Ingredients: *1 Quart Vegetable Stock (approx 32-36 cubes)*
Potatoes - 5 to 6 large spuds (peeled, cut & boiled)
Carrots - 3 to 4 large (peeled and diced or sliced)
Celery - 2 to 3 large stalks (diced)
Leeks - 1 large (finely sliced)
Onion - 1 medium (diced)
Garlic - 2 to 3 large pieces (diced)
Butter - 6 to 8 Tbs. depending upon
        amount of potatoes used
Milk - 3 Tbs (optional)
Salt and pepper - to taste

- *Mash boiled potatoes with 4 to 6 Tbs of butter, add 3 Tbs milk if preferred. Set aside.*

- *Over medium heat, melt 2 Tbs butter in skillet, add garlic, onion, celery, leeks and saute untiled browned (approximately 15 minutes)*

- *In soup pan, heat 1 quart of vegetable stock to under boiling. Add carrots.*

- *When celery, onion, leeks and garlic are browned, add to soup pot and then add in mashed potatoes, stir until combined. Salt and pepper to taste.*

- *Heat to boiling, reduce heat and simmer for 10 minutes. Then serve.*

PB & J

Peanut butter and jelly sandwiches are my favorite. Especially grilled! Nothing like it in the whole world. But almost every jelly and jam on the market contains *pectin*, a source of MSG I don't tolerate well at all. To get around that, we've begun to make our own jam. Here's a recipe for strawberry.

- *Wash all fruit (Organic varieties preferred.)*
- *Use appropriately sized sauce pan (non-aluminum)*
- *Use sterilized glass sealing jars*
- *Makes approximately 2 quarts*

Ingredients: *4 lbs. fresh strawberries - wash and hull*
2 1/2 lbs sugar - (cane sugar)

Dry berries and mash. Combine in sauce pan with sugar over medium heat. Bring to a boil and then cook over low heat for 30 to 40 minutes, stirring often. Pour into sterilized jars, seal and store in the refrigerator.

Spaghetti Sauce & Alphabets ...

Ingredients: *Organic Tomato Sauce - 8 oz can*
Organic Tomato Paste - 5 oz can
Organic Alphabet Noodles - 1 cup
Asiago or Romano cheese - 1/4 cup shredded
(optional)*

Boil noodles until tender and strain. Place in sauce pan and add tomato sauce and paste, heat, stirring occasionally. Add Asiago or Romano cheese (optional)*

* may be processed with enzymes

Banana Bread ...

- *Though contrary to the practices of "good food combining", we like our banana bread. It's great to put into lunch boxes or keep in the refrigerator at work for quick bites. It's both breakfast, snack and dessert!*
- *Use non-aluminum cake or loaf pans. Makes one pan loaf.*

Ingredients: *Bananas - 3 or 4 medium, ripe*
Egg - 2
Butter - 1/3 cup, softened
Water - 1/3 cup
Sugar - 1 cup
Unenriched Flour - 1 2/3 cups
Baking Soda - 1 tsp
Baking powder - 1/4 tsp
Salt - 1/2 tsp
Nuts - 1/2 cup chopped (optional)

Heat oven to 350°. Only grease the bottom of your pan.

Mix sugar and butter in bowl and stir in eggs until blended. Mash bananas and add with water, beat until well blended together. Add baking soda & powder, salt and nuts (if preferred - walnuts, pecans, etc). Pour into your loaf pan and bake about 50 to 60 minutes for loaf pan and approximately 35 to 40 minutes for shallow pan. A toothpick stuck into the center of the loaf should come out cleanly when done. Cool completely before cutting.

Salad Dressings & Condiments

We love our salads! Big, colorful chunky salads with lots of variety and taste. Bottled dressings are a bit of a pain though. Most brands, even organic and "natural"and especially "fat free" varieties, contain xanthum gum, carreegnan or other "biochemically engineered fats and thickeners" that contain MSG, so, again, we opt to make our own.

Any vinegar or soy sauce naturally adds a bit of risk to any meal plan. Vinegars are fermented liquids that can hasten the fermentation (breakdown) of proteins they come in contact with like cheese used in a salad, meats used with a marinade, soy with fish and rice.

If you are just starting your elimination, try eating salads without dressings first, then add oils, lemon, herbs and then add vinegars and soy back into your diet as part of your plan. Remember to note what brand and type you were using (white, cider, wine, other) and any negative reactions.

- *Use good quality vinegars without added sulfite or other ingredients such as sulfur (Organic varieties preferred.)*

- *Wine vinegars may have yeasts, tannin and sulfates added.*

- *Commercial buttermilk is often made by the use of enzymes which may increase the potential for a MSG sensitivity reaction. Use with caution.*

- *Most catsup and mayonnaise also contains ingredients on our **Hidden Sources** list. Check for organic, vegetable based products in your health food stores or try the recipes we have here.*

Hot & Sour Bacon Dressing

- *Great over spinach, walnuts & gorganzola cheese or with mixed greens or dandelions with pinion nuts*

- *This makes an interesting glaze for baked chicken or pork*

- *I would use caution with this recipe if you are in your beginning phases of elimination or extremely sensitive to MSG*

Ingredients: Bacon - 4 large slices (well marbled)
                    use brands without additives and preservatives
                Egg - 1 beaten
                Unenriched, Unsifted Flour - 3 tsps
                Water - 1 1/2 cups
                Vinegar - 2 Tbs (Cider, yellow or white)
                Salt - 1/2 tsp

Fry bacon crisp, put aside to drain and cool. Pour off bacon grease except for 2 Tbs. which you will leave in skillet. Blend flour and salt to the fat over low heat, stirring constantly. Add water gradually and then stir in egg and vinegar. Continue to stir over low heat until mixture thickens. Use immediately. You can store remainder in refrigerator, heat and serve later.

Grandma's French Dressing

- *We use a dressing cruet we have, but any sealable glass jar or container will do for preparation and storage.*

Ingredients:		
Sugar - 1 tsp		Salt - 1 tsp
Pepper - 1/4 tsp		Dry Mustard - 1/4 tsp
Paprika - 1 tsp		Garlic - to taste
Wine Vinegar - 1 oz.		Vegetable Oil - 3/4 cup

Combine dry ingredients, then add to container with oil and vinegar. Shake well and serve.

"Mayo"...

Ingredients: 1 1/2 cups salad oil (safflower or canola)
Egg - 1 large
Vinegar - 2 Tbs
Salt - 1 tps
Sugar - 1 tsp
Dry Mustard - 1 tsp
Salt, paprika, pepper to taste

Combine salt, sugar and dry mustard in small mixer bowl. Add vinegar and the egg and beat until thoroughly blended. Continue to beat mixture while slowly pouring the salad oil in until it reaches a desired consistency. Add additional spices to taste.

Store in the refrigerator (approximately 5-7 days) in air-tight container.

Mom's Mayo Dressing

• We usual make this up as needed.

Ingredients: Lemon - 1 tsp   Salt & Pepper - to taste
Celery Seed - 1/4 tsp   Garlic - to taste
Mayo - 2 Tbsp

Combine ingredients and serve with greens and mixed raw vegetables or as a "dip" for celery, carrots or other vegetable finger foods.

Catsup ...

- *If you can't find a commercial brand of catsup you tolerate, try making your own.*
- *This recipe will yield approximately 2 pints of catsup*
- *You will need sealing canning jars*

Ingredients: Tomatoes - 8 pounds (we like to use roma)
Onion - 1 medium (chopped)
Green Pepper - 1 cup (chopped)
Sugar - 1 cup
White vinegar - 1 cup
Cayenne pepper - 1/4 tsp
Cloves - 1 1/2 tsp (whole)
Cinnamon - 1 1/2 inch stick or approx 1 tsp powder
Celery Seed - 1 tsp
Salt - 4 tsp (then to taste)

Wash and core tomatoes. Cut into quarters and let drain for 15 minutes. Combine tomatoes, cayenne, celery seed, onion and green pepper in large kettle pot over medium heat. Bring to a boil and cook for 40 to 50 minutes. Stir occasionally, making sure the ingredients don't stick. If this occurs, lower your heat.

Take finished product and put through a course sieve or food mill. (I have an old colander with holes just small enough to keep seeds from getting through that I use. I put an equal sized kettle pot in the sink, put the colander inside of it and strain the tomatoes right into the next pot.) Discard remaining seeds and skin.

Add vinegar, sugar and salt to the tomatoes and bring to a boil over medium heat. Reduce heat and simmer until it thickens, stirring often. When it reaches a nice consistency, pour into hot glass canning jars. Remember to leave "head space" - about 2 inches will do, adjust lids and process in boiling water bath for 10 minutes. Refrigerate.

Order a copy of The Feel Good Handbook for friend or family member!

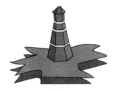

The LightHouse Press

You can: *5/00*

Call 888-298-1500 and order over the phone ...

•or•

Visit our website at

www.thelighthousepress.com or *www.msgfree.com*

•or•

You can photo copy or tear out & mail in this completed order form to:

The LightHouse Press
3555 W. El Camino Real, #301
San Mateo, CA 94403

Bill To: _
Address: _
City, State & Zip: _
Day Time Phone: _

Ship To: _
Address: _
City, State Zip: _

The Feel Good Handbook
(ISBN 0-9662169-9-7)   ____ X $14.95 each _____
California Residents, please add 7.5% Sales Tax: _____
Shipping & Handling (US Post) $ 3.00
                              Total Due: _____

Credit Card # _
Exp Date: _
Account Name: _
Billing Zip Code: _
Signature: _